CHINESE HEALING SECRETS

Bill Schoenbart, L.Ac.
Consultant: Ellen Shefi, L.Ac., LMT

Publications International, Ltd.

Bill Schoenbart is licensed in both herbal medicine and acupuncture and has an M.A. in Chinese medicine. He is a member of the faculty of the American School of Herbalism and of the Hawaii School of Traditional Chinese Medicine. He is editor of *The Way of Chinese Herbs* and *Biomagnetic and Herbal Therapy*.

Ellen Shefi is a licensed massage technician, licensed acupuncturist, and registered dietician. She operates a private acupuncture practice, has assisted in developing acupuncture protocol, and has contributed to a national research project funded by the National Institutes of Health Office of Alternative Medicine. She is a member of the American Association of Acupuncture and Oriental Medicine, the American Herb Association, and the Oregon Acupuncture Association.

Illustrations: **Yoshi Miyaki; Susan Spellman.**

Front cover photo: **Stephen Simpson/FPG International.**

Picture credits: **Cathy Wilkinson Barash:** 97; **Custom Medical Stock Photo:** 8, 55, 153; Amethyst: table of contents (right center & bottom right), 99, 106; Eric Nelson: 122; Vincent Zuber: 35; **Marnae Ergil, Wind Horse:** 113; **FPG International:** 100% Rag Productions: 109; Adamsmith: 43; Tony Anderson: 28; Frank Cezus: 66; Willard Clay: 69; Jim Cummins: 40, 59; Steve Hix: 76; Spencer Jones: 18; Jeff Kaufman: 94, 158; Dick Luria: 33; Christian Michaels: 114; Keren Su: 192; Joyce Tenneson: 24; Tom Wilson: 85; **Gerry Gropp/Sipa Press:** 16, 117; **International Stock:** Jim Cambon: 146; Al Clayton: 88; Warren Faidley: 21; Vincent Graziani: 62; Kit Luce: 145, 157; Lou Manna: 91; John Michael: 52; Valder Tormey: 31; Michael Ventura: 149; Caroline Wood: 128; **Postive Images:** Patricia J. Bruno: 5, 104; Arleen Lorrance: 50, 57, 126, 142; **Rainbow:** Dan McCoy: table of contents (top right), 37, 46; Coco McCoy: 81; Frank Siteman: 74, 78; **SuperStock:** table of contents (top left, left center & bottom left), 9, 10, 14; Lucia Gallery, New, York City: title page, 135; **Mark Taylor:** 25.

Manufactured in China

8 7 6 5 4 3 2 1

ISBN: 0-7853-2433-X

Library of Congress Catalog Card Number: 97-67522

Note: Neither the Editors of Consumer Guide™ and Publications International, Ltd., nor the author, consultant, editors, or publisher take responsibility for any possible consequences from any treatment, procedure, exercise, dietary modification, action, or application of medication or preparation by any person reading or following the information in this book. The publication of this book does not constitute the practice of medicine, and this book does not attempt to replace your physician or your pharmacist. Before undertaking any course of treatment, the author, consultant, editors, and publisher advise the reader to check with a physician or other health care provider.

CONTENTS

INTRODUCTION

As the late afternoon sun sinks behind the mountain, a silent figure walks slowly along the slope. Occasionally he kneels on the ground, gazing intently at a plant that has caught his attention. After careful consideration, he digs up some roots and washes them off in a stream. Carefully planting some of the plant's ripe berries, he heads up the trail at a brisk pace. Home is another 15 miles away, in a fertile river valley on the other side of the mountain. Chewing on one of the man-shaped roots, he doesn't seem bothered by the difficult trek that lies

ahead of him. After all, he's been taking this trip every autumn for the last 75 years! Breathing in a deep meditation, he feels his energy level build as he walks along. Dark clouds threaten snow on the pass, but he feels confident that

Even with the development of modern medicine, millions of people around the world still turn to herbs for healing.

the breathing exercises and the "man roots" will keep him warm. Satisfied that his inner climate is in harmony with the mountain weather, he heads for his home to help the villagers put up food and medicines for the long winter ahead.

When he finally reaches his home village the next morning, a group of children rushes up to greet him. When he slides his travel pack off his shoulder, they jump with glee, knowing that he has brought them some treats from the mountains. Reaching into his sack, he hands each child a sweet yellow root, and they run off to chew on their coveted snacks. Their mother nods in approval, knowing that the "sweet root" will ward off the sore throats that are so common with the coming of autumn weather.

Arriving at his simple hut, he finds a group of villagers waiting. An elderly woman walks up to him, worried that she can't seem to stay warm in the colder weather. Gently holding her wrist, he notices that her pulse is faint and difficult to find. He has already observed that her face and tongue are pale; when she reports that she wakes up throughout the night to urinate, his diagnosis is confirmed. "Not enough yang in the kidneys," he exclaims. He reaches into his medicine bag for a cigar-shaped cylinder of dried herbs and slowly lights it in the communal fire. Gently swirling the smoldering herbs over points below her knees and low back, he instructs an apprentice to prepare an herbal formula for her. The woman is confident that the formula will work—her great-grandmother used the very same herbs when she experienced a similar condition. She remembers it well: When she was a little girl, she asked granny for a sip of her tea. Her grandmother simply laughed and said to her, "Sorry, little one. Your yang is too strong. This tea is for old people." Almost a century later, already feeling better from the burning herbs, she looks forward to drinking the brew being

The burning of "moxa"—made from the mugwort herb—near specific points is an ancient and trusted Chinese healing technique.

Chinese Healing Secrets

prepared for her. One by one, the villagers approach the old herbalist, explaining their symptoms to him. In each case, he feels the pulses on both their wrists and looks carefully at their tongue. His diagnoses sound like weather reports: cold and damp; wind with heat; excessive heat leading to dryness. He is a Taoist; his world view consists of an unbroken unity between human beings and the universe that they inhabit.

This perception is at the root of traditional Chinese medicine: The individual (microcosm) is viewed as an integral part of the forces of nature (macrocosm). By careful observation of nature, Taoist sages were able to perceive patterns common to both the external environment and the internal climate of the human body. Over a period of thousands of years, the cumulative observations of sages all over China led to an intricate system of diagnosis and healing.

Even after the development of modern scientific medicine, this ancient practice is still used by millions of people all over the world. For some ailments, such as chronic degenerative disease and viral infections, traditional Chinese medicine is superior to modern medicine. In other areas, such as life-threatening infections or severe physical trauma, there is no substitute for Western medicine. In modern Chinese hospitals, there is no antagonism between modern and ancient medicine. Both systems are practiced, often by the same people. Cancer patients, for example, might undergo surgery or chemotherapy in order to remove or reduce a tumor and then receive herbal formulas to restore their blood count to normal and help them recover their strength. Another example of the blending of the two systems of medicine is the use of acupuncture anesthesia, which lessens the danger of drug reactions during surgery. In thyroid operations, the parathyroid glands are often accidentally removed. When acupuncture anesthesia is used, the patient feels an electrical sensation when the scalpel gets too close to the parathyroid; his instant feedback prevents the inadvertent removal of an important gland. Thus, the wisdom of the past has been integrated with the practices of the present.

The practice of herbal medicine in China has come a long way since the days of the old herbalist. Ginseng, known in China as ren shen, or "man root," was the man-shaped root that helped the old herbalist over the mountain pass. Although the old man knew from experience that it strengthened his yang and qi, modern research confirms his early observations. Ginseng has been found to enhance the body's ability to adapt to stress, reduce fatigue, and stimulate the immune system. Similarly, the sweet root that he gave out to the children was licorice, or gan cao

Ancient Chinese healers knew that licorice could soothe inflamed throats.

("sweet herb"). The villagers knew from experience that it would support the children's qi and soothe "fire toxicity" (sore throats). Thousands of years later, pharmacologic research finds that licorice strengthens the adrenal glands and has powerful anti-inflammatory activity, making it effective in treating all kinds of inflammation as well as ulcers, asthma, and tuberculosis. The ancient remedies have more than withstood the tests of time—they have passed the tests of modern medicine.

Chinese Healing Secrets offers an introduction to the theories and practice of traditional Chinese medicine. The book opens with a brief look at the history and development of traditional Chinese medicine. Chapters 2 through 4 present the Taoist theory of the human body, beginning with the theory of yin and yang and how events in nature are reflected within the human body. Each subsequent chapter builds on this basic Taoist theory. Chapters 5 through 7 explain how to recognize patterns of disharmony. Interestingly, learning to recognize patterns of disharmony in the human body is much like learning to understand weather patterns. Once you understand the patterns of disharmony, you can understand how they can be treated with the various methods described in Chapter 8. Chapter 9 gives you helpful advice on choosing a practitioner of traditional Chinese medicine.

The second part of the book lists common ailments, outlines how a practitioner of traditional Chinese medicine might treat these ailments, and describes patent medicines—herbal remedies you can use at home to treat conditions ranging from the common cold to insomnia.

While some of its treatments may seem quite foreign to Westerners, traditional Chinese medicine is moving into the medical mainstream.

The remarkable system of traditional Chinese medicine is one of China's great gifts to humanity. Practically unknown in the West until the 1970s, the secrets of Chinese healing are rapidly becoming part of the mainstream of medicine. The purpose of this book is to share this vast wealth of knowledge and empower you to begin using this ancient wisdom in your own life.

CHAPTER 1:
The History of Traditional Chinese Medicine

Archeological excavations reveal that human beings lived in China more than a million years ago. These primitive people spent most of their time on basic survival: hunting, locating and preparing plants for food, building shelters, and defending themselves. It's easy to imagine that over time, they'd have sampled most of the local plants in their search for food. In time, an oral record evolved that identified those plants that made good food, those that were useful for building, those that had an effect on illness, and those that were poisonous. Through trial and error, a primitive form of herbal medicine and dietary therapy was taking shape in China.

The use of plants for health and healing has been a mainstay of Chinese medicine for thousands of years.

Fire also played a central role in their lives as a source of warmth, fuel, and light. As they huddled around fires, it was only natural that our ancestors would discover the healing powers of heat. Those powers would have been especially evident for cold, damp ailments such as arthritis, for which heat provides immediate relief. This was the origin of the art of moxibustion, the therapeutic application of heat to treat a wide variety of conditions.

These ancient people must have experienced a variety of injuries during their rugged lives. A natural reaction to pain is to rub or press on the affected area. This hands-on therapy gradually evolved into a system of therapeutic manipulation. People discovered that pressing on certain points on the body had wide-ranging effects. They began to use pieces of sharpened bone or stone to enhance the sensation, and acupuncture was born.

WRITTEN HISTORY

The development of a written record of Chinese medicine has evolved mostly over the last 3,000 years. Archeological digs from the Shang Dynasty (1,000 B.C.) have revealed medical writings inscribed on divination bones: Early shamans, mostly women, used scapula bones to perform divination rites; later these bones were also used for writing. The discovery in 1973 of 11 medical texts written on silk has shed some light on the sophisticated practices of that early period of Chinese history. Dated to 168 B.C., the texts discuss diet, exercise, moxibustion, and herbal therapy. Liberally mixed with shamanistic magic, an extensive text, *Prescriptions for Fifty-two Ailments*, describes the pharmacologic effects of herbs and foods. Also dating from about this time is the legend of Shen Nong, the

Ancient Chinese healers were quite sophisticated in their use of natural materials, taking advantage of the healing energy in plants, animals, and minerals in their prescriptions.

Emperor of Agriculture, who tasted 100 herbs daily to assess their qualities. (He is said to have been poisoned many times in the course of his investigations.) The book that is attributed to him is known as the *Classic of the Agriculture Emperor's Materia Medica*. It lists 365 medicines, comprising 252 plants, 67 animals, and 46 minerals. Tao Hong-Jing, the editor of the version of Shen Nong's materia medica in use today, divided the herbs into three classes. The upper-class herbs are non-toxic tonics that strengthen and nourish the body, the middle-grade herbs are tonics with therapeutic qualities, and the lower grade consists of herbs that treat disease or possess some toxicity. This classification system gives a glimpse into an important principle in traditional Chinese medicine: It is better to strengthen the body and prevent disease than to fight illness once it has already taken hold. Ignoring preventive health care and waiting to treat disease was considered as foolish as waiting until you are thirsty to dig a well.

By A.D. 400, the basic foundations of traditional Chinese medicine had been put into written form. By this time, most of the magical aspects of medicine had been left behind; there was an increasing belief in the powers of nature to heal disease. The most important book compiled between 300 B.C. and A.D. 400 is *The Yellow Emperor's Inner Classic (Huang Di Nei Jing)*. The work is purported to be a series of conversations between the Yellow Emperor, Huang Di, and his minister, Qi Bo, although many historians believe it is a compilation of all the medical knowledge of that period. The work is divided into two books: *Simple Questions* and *Spiritual Axis*. The first book deals with general theoretical principles, while the second more specifically describes the principles of acupuncture and the treatment of disease. Remarkably, this ancient work is still valid; it forms the foundation for the contemporary practice of traditional Chinese medicine. For example, the *Nei Jing* states that cold diseases should be treated with hot herbs, and hot diseases should be treated with cold herbs. This principle is still followed today in clinical practice. Hot, inflammatory infections are treated with cold herbs such as honeysuckle flowers or *Coptis* root; cold, debilitating conditions such as chronic fatigue are treated with warm, stimulating herbs such as ginseng or *Astragalus* roots. Modern research has confirmed that these plants contain constituents with strong pharmacologic effects on these specific conditions.

By the second century A.D., physicians all over China were compiling writings of the latest discoveries in acupuncture and herbal medicine. It was during this time that the famous physician Hua Tuo wrote about herbal anesthesia. Although his formula for the anesthetic has been lost, his unique system of acupuncture points is still in use. He was also a pioneer in recommending exercise as a method of maintaining wellness. He is quoted as saying "a running stream never goes bad," meaning exercise moves qi and prevents the stagnation that leads to disease. Another pioneer of the time was Zhang Zhongjing, who wrote *Treatise on Febrile and Mis-*

One of the oldest-known Chinese medical texts lists more than 365 medicines for healing. Some of the herbs prescribed in the text, such as ginger, cinnamon, and ma huang, are still used in Chinese medicine today.

cellaneous Diseases after witnessing an epidemic that ravaged his city and killed most of his relatives. This highly regarded physician developed a system of diagnosis so sophisticated that it is used by practitioners in modern hospitals 1,700 years after his death.

Progress of Medicine in China

Between the 2nd and 5th centuries (A.D.), China experienced a period marked by war and political turmoil. One of the ironies of war is that it has a tendency to lead to advances in medicine. The periodic times of unrest in Chinese history, such as this, were no exception, as the increased need for practical, convenient, effective remedies led to further developments in medical treatment. During this time, Ge Hong wrote *Prescriptions for Emergencies* in order to spread the knowledge of acupuncture and moxibustion to the masses. Around A.D. 650, Sun Simiao compiled *Prescriptions Worth A Thousand Gold*, which integrated the clinical experiences of the different schools of acupuncture at that time. During the Tang Dynasty (618–907 A.D.), China's Imperial Medical Bureau established departments of Acupuncture, Pharmacology, and Medical Specialties, and numerous additional treatises and compilations of medical

The art of the traditional Chinese medicine practitioner is based on accumulated knowledge and experience passed down through the ages.

knowledge and experience were prepared.

In the Five Dynasties period (907–1368 A.D.), advancements in printing techniques led to a dramatic increase in the publication of medical texts. One of the important books of the period was *Canon on the Origin of Acupuncture and Moxibustion*, in which Wang Zhizhong incorporated the clinical experiences of the practitioners of folk medicine. During the

Ming Dynasty (1368–1644), many medical specialists compiled the works of their forebears, further expanding the extensive base of medical knowledge. The most famous physician of the period was Li Shi Zheng (1518–1593), a kind and generous healer who did not accept payment for his services. After reviving the son of a prince from a coma, he was appointed court physician and served in the Imperial Academy of Medicine. His most incredible achievement was his 40-year effort in writing the *Ben Cao Gong Mu* (*General Catalog of Herbs*), a monumental work published after his death. Consisting of 52 volumes at the time of its printing, the *Ben Cao Gong Mu* remains an important reference for traditional Chinese herbalists.

RECENT HISTORY

The integration of new techniques with ancient understanding continued until the 19th century, when the Opium War of 1840 turned China into a semicolonial society. Western colonial powers derided traditional medicine as primitive and outdated. The Communist party came to power in the mid-20th century, bringing much turmoil to China; however, the Communists saw the need to promote traditional Chinese medicine to avoid dependence on the West. A great need for traditional doctors arose since there were far too few Western-trained physicians to serve the huge population: only 10,000 Western-trained doctors were available to serve 400 million people. Traditional Chinese medicine began a course of revival that continues today.

Many Western-trained physicians and scientists in China started to conduct research on acupuncture, moxibustion, and herbal medicine, and a gradual integration of the two systems began. In 1945, an acupuncture clinic opened in a Western hospital in China for the first time. Since then, traditional Chinese medicine and Western medicine have been practiced side by side in Chinese hospitals, sometimes by a physician who has been trained in both fields. For example, a cancer patient might receive radiation to treat a tumor then be sent to the herbal department for formulas to strengthen his immune system and normalize his blood count.

Since the 1970s, Chinese hospitals have trained students from more than 100 countries in the principles of traditional medicine. Interest in traditional Chinese medicine was sparked in the United States in the early 1970s when *The New York Times* reporter James Reston experienced an acute appendicitis attack while in China. His report of receiving acupuncture to relieve his postoperative abdominal pain brought an awareness of this system of healing to the general public.

Today in China, many medical practitioners have been trained in the methods of both Western medicine and traditional Chinese medicine, allowing patients to reap the benefits of both systems.

Since then, acupuncture and herbal medicine have gradually taken hold in North America. With more than 10,000 practitioners and an increasing number of schools of traditional Chinese medicine, this ancient system has taken its well-deserved place in the Western world.

CHAPTER 2:
The Theory
of Yin and Yang

Through patient observation of the forces of nature, the Taoists who developed the system of traditional Chinese medicine saw the universe as a unified field, constantly moving and changing while maintaining its oneness. This constant state of change was explained through the theory of yin and yang, which first appeared in written form around

The Chinese character for Yin.

The Chinese character for Yang.

700 B.C. in the I Ching ("Book of Changes"). According to the theory, nature expresses itself in an endless cycle of polar opposites such as day and night, moisture and dryness, heat and cold, and activity and rest. Yin phenomena are those that exhibit the nurturing qualities of darkness, rest, moisture, cold, and structure. Its Chinese character depicts the shady side of a hill. Yang phenomena have qualities of energy such as light, activity, dryness, heat, and function. Its Chinese character represents the sunny side of a hill. Everything in nature exhibits varying combinations of both yin and yang. For example, the morning fog (yin) is dissipated by the heat of the sun (yang); the forest fire (yang) is extinguished by the rainstorm (yin); the darkness of night (yin) is replaced by the light of day (yang). Any phenomenon within nature can be understood in relation to another; one will always be yin or yang in comparison with the other.

Some of the basic principles of yin and yang:

- **Everything in nature can be expressed as the opposition of yin and yang.** This is the energizing force of all aspects of nature. It is dynamic and the basic foundation for change in nature. Yin and yang are also relative terms: A forest fire is more yang than a campfire; a campfire is more yang than a spark. Nothing is purely yin or yang; it is always a matter of comparison.

The opposition of yin and yang is the energizing force in the world.

- **Yin and yang are interdependent.** Even though yin and yang are opposites, one has no meaning without the other. For example, day would have no meaning without night; heat cannot be understood without knowing what cold feels like; fever and chills can't be determined without experiencing the normal body temperature.

- **Yin creates yang; yang creates yin.** Numerous examples of this principle can be seen in nature. For example, on a hot summer day (yang), there is a sudden thunderstorm (yin). A person may get symptoms of chills and a runny nose (yin) that turn into a fever with a sore throat (yang). A hyperactive child runs around frantically (yang), then suddenly falls asleep (yin).

- **Yin and yang mutually control each other.** This is the basic mechanism of balance in nature and the human body. When the body gets overheated from exercise, the pores open and sweating lowers the temperature. When the body gets too cold due to exposure, the muscles shiver to generate heat.

Since the Taoists believe that everything is part of the oneness of the universe, they make no distinction between the external forces of nature and the internal processes of the human body, believing that "the macrocosm exists within the microcosm." In other words, any process or change that can be witnessed in nature can also be seen in the body. For example, a person who eats cold food (yin) on a cold, damp day (yin) may experience excessive mucus (yin). Similarly, a person who performs strenuous activity (yang) on a hot day (yang) might experience dehydration with a fever (yang). Some of the traditional diagnoses sound like weather reports, such as "wind and cold with dampness" (a yin condition) or a "deficiency of moisture leading to fire" (a yang pattern). These diagnostic descriptions illustrate the principle that the body experiences the same fluctuations of yin and yang as the environment.

The internal organs also have their own balance of yin and yang. Yin functions tend to be nourishing, cooling, building, and relaxing and relate to the structure, or substance, of the organs. Yang qualities tend to be energizing, warming, consuming, and stimulating and relate to the functional activity of the organs. For example, the kidneys are considered the source of yin (water) and yang (fire, or metabolism) for the entire body. If the kidney yin is deficient or depleted, a person can experience hot flashes and night sweats, as occurs in menopause when estrogen (yin) levels decline. This is due to insufficient moisture (yin) to keep the metabolic fire (yang), which keeps the body warm, under control. Think of running a car engine with insufficient oil; the engine will overheat due to a deficiency of this yin-like lubricant. A deficiency of kidney yang produces such symptoms as cold hands and feet and a general lack of vitality. These symptoms, which often occur with age, are due to insufficient metabolic fire (yang) to infuse the entire body with energy and warmth, dispersing cold and fatigue (yin).

The curve in the traditional yin-yang symbol represents the ever-changing balance between yin and yang; the small circles show that each contains elements of the other.

Traditional Chinese medicine applies this ancient theory of yin and yang in clinical practice. In the case of kidney yin deficiency, the therapeutic principle is to tonify (fortify) the yin and sedate the hyperactive yang. This is achieved with a classic formula known as "Rehmannia Teapills," which contain three herbs that nourish the kidneys' yin and three herbs that clear the heat that arises from the lack of the cooling and moistening yin functions. In kidney yang deficiency, similar herbs are used to nourish the kidney, with the addition of warming metabolic stimulants such as *Aconite* root and cinnamon bark. Since all the organs have similar yin and yang aspects, it is possible to monitor and adjust the yin and yang levels of all parts of the body, maintaining a high level of vitality and preventing disease. This is achieved not only with herbs but with changes in diet and lifestyle. In this way, the ancient observations of the Taoists have practical applications in our own quest for wellness.

CHAPTER 3:
The Vital Substances

In traditional Chinese medicine, the body and mind are inseparable. Composed of a number of vital substances—qi (pronounced chee), blood, essence, and body fluids—the body and mind express their qualities through the functions of the internal organs. Ranging from tangible, visible substances to subtle, intangible forces, these basic elements of the body/mind are responsible for all aspects of human life—physical, mental, emotional, and spiritual. Their intimate involvement in human activity makes them an essential part of physiology, and recognition and understanding of them are an essential part of diagnosis.

QI

Although qi plays a central role in traditional Chinese medicine, it is extremely difficult to define. It is best to understand it in terms of its functions and activities, where it is more readily perceived. Situated somewhere between matter and energy, qi has the qualities of both. It

The power of qi can be observed in the fallen trees and damaged buildings left after a thunderstorm has passed through.

has substance without structure, and it possesses energy qualities but can't be measured. It is the fundamental power underlying all the activities of nature as well as the vital life force of the human body. For example, the force of a thunderstorm can be understood in terms of its qi: The power of qi can be observed in the fallen trees and buildings in the storm's aftermath. Similarly, the strength of the digestive organs can be determined in relation to their qi by evaluating the appetite, color of the tongue, strength of the pulse, and the body's response to nutrition.

The flow of qi through the body occurs within a closed system of channels, or meridians. There are 12 major meridians, and they correspond to the 12 organ systems: six yin organs and six yang organs. Traditional organ theory pairs yin and yang organs according to their structure and function and the interconnection of their meridians. For a full discussion of yin and yang organs and their functions, see Chapter 4, "The Internal Organs." In addition, eight extra meridians are interconnected with all the channels. This network of meridians allows the qi, or life force, to reach all the tissues and organs, providing nourishment, warmth, and energy to all parts of the body. The flow of qi travels from channel to channel, passing through all the meridians every 24 hours. For example, the flow of qi in the heart meridian is strongest between the hours of 11 a.m. and 1 p.m. From there, the qi flows into the meridian of the small intestine, staying there until 3 p.m., at which time the flow passes into the bladder meridian. In this way, qi passes through all the major

Flow of Qi

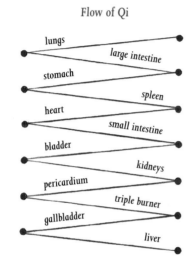

lungs
large intestine
stomach
spleen
heart
small intestine
bladder
kidneys
pericardium
triple burner
gallbladder
liver

Qi passes through all the major meridians and their corresponding organs every day.

meridians and their corresponding organs every day. Although the meridians are deep within the body, points along them are accessible from the surface of the skin. It is the manipulation of these points by means of pressure, heat, or needles that is the basis for acupressure, moxibustion, and acupuncture, respectively. The qi that flows through the meridians can be manipulated at the acupuncture points, bringing healing energy to organs that need it and moving energy away from areas that are impaired due to stagnation of qi.

FUNCTIONS OF QI

Although many types of specialized qi exist in the body, such as those associated with a particular organ, all varieties share some basic functions. These functions are as follows:

- Transformation: Qi transforms one type of substance into another. Spleen qi transforms food into qi and blood the body can use; kidney qi transforms fluids into pure essence and waste water; lung qi transforms air into the energy to sustain life.
- Movement: All movement is accompanied by its own qi, including growth and development and even walking, breathing, and thinking. Qi moves the blood through the vessels, giving rise to the saying, "Qi is the commander of the blood."
- Protection: Qi protects the body from attacks by disease-causing organisms. Therefore, if a person's qi is weak, that person may experience frequent illnesses.
- Retention: Qi keeps the organs in their proper place, keeps blood within the vessels, and keeps body fluids inside the body. Deficiency of qi can lead to sagging organs (prolapse), bleeding disorders, and excessive sweating or urination.

- Warming: The yang aspect of kidney qi keeps the entire body warm; when it is deficient, chronic cold extremities and decreased function in all activities that require warmth, such as digestion, can occur.

TYPES OF QI

Chinese medicine traditionally divides qi into various types, depending on its source and function. The original source of this life force is a person's parents, and the qi inherited from them is known as prenatal qi. Prenatal qi, the basic constitution of a human being, depends on genetics and the quality of the parents' lives at the time of conception and during pregnancy. This qi is the person's heritage, and it cannot be replenished; however, healthy lifestyle, diet, and breathing practices can conserve prenatal qi and slow down its depletion. Preservation of prenatal qi is one of the most important contributions of traditional Chinese medicine. It enables a person who is sickly and weak to live a life of health and vitality. The process involves a simultaneous conservation of prenatal qi with practices that enhance the formation of postnatal qi.

The qi a person inherits from their parents is called prenatal qi. Prenatal qi is a person's heritage, and it can't be replenished, although a healthy lifestyle can slow its depletion.

Postnatal qi, or acquired qi, is derived from the digestion of food and extracted from the air we breathe. Combined with prenatal qi, it forms the totality of the body's power to perform all the vital processes of life. One of the functions of the lungs is to extract qi from air and incorporate it into the storehouse of postnatal qi. The strength of postnatal qi depends on a number of factors: the strength of lung qi, the quality of the air, and the performance of breathing exercises such as qi gong,

which enhances the lungs' ability to extract qi from air. When lung qi is deficient, a person can experience symptoms of fatigue, shortness of breath, pallor, and frequent colds. The other factor in building strong postnatal qi is the quality of the food we eat and the strength of our digestive organs, especially the spleen. When spleen qi is weak, symptoms of fatigue, lack of appetite, sluggishness, and loose stools can occur. When the diet lacks essential nutrients and variety, the extraction of qi is impaired even if spleen qi is strong. People accustomed to eating fresh organic fruits, vegetables, and

Herbs that tonify lung and spleen qi, along with breathing exercises such as qi gong, can increase the accumulation of postnatal qi, which can help overcome the effects of weak prenatal qi.

whole grains will often experience this when circumstances force them to eat denatured, refined, pesticide-laden foods: Inevitably, they notice their energy level drops. Recent research has confirmed that organically grown produce has significantly higher levels of nutrients.

When both spleen qi and lung qi are strong, and the quality of our air and food are high, postnatal qi can grow. Herbs that tonify lung and spleen qi, along with breathing practices such as qi gong, further increase the accumulation of postnatal qi. In this way, even a person with a weak inherited constitution (prenatal qi) can experience a life of health and vitality.

The totality of qi that results from the combination of prenatal and postnatal qi is known as true qi. Responsible for all the functions of the body, true qi takes different forms. From the clinical perspective, two of these forms of qi are especially significant: nutritive qi and protective qi.

Nutritive qi circulates in the meridians and nourishes the organs. Acupuncture manipulates this qi to affect organ function. Specific points along the meridians are needled, pressed, or warmed (by means of moxibustion) to achieve specific effects in the organs. For example, a point below the knee is manipulated traditionally to treat appendicitis, often eliminating the symptoms when the condition is caught before infection sets in. When a Chinese surgeon performing appendectomies needled this point on his patients, he found that the intestines contracted rhythmically on either side of the appendix. This demonstrates how the power of qi can be observed, even when it is difficult to understand exactly how it is working.

The other important subdivision of true qi is protective qi, or wei qi. Believed to flow between the skin and muscles, wei qi is responsible for defending the body from external pathogens that attack the body. Although first described thousands of years ago, wei qi accurately describes the body's immune system. Research has confirmed that herbs traditionally used to tonify wei qi, such as *Astragalus* root (huang qi), have a powerful effect in strengthening the body's resistance to disease and increasing immune function. Certain acupuncture points, such as Stomach 36 (Zusanli) and Large Intestine 4 (Hegu), have similar effects on immune function.

DISORDERS OF QI

Chinese medicine seeks to ensure that the levels, direction, and flow of qi are all appropriate for their particular organs. The various disorders of qi that can occur involve deficiency, sinking, stagnation, or incorrect movement of qi. The symptoms of qi deficiency are common to all the types of qi disorders: fatigue, pallor, and lethargy. When the qi of an organ is deficient, the specific functions of that organ are also impaired. For example, the spleen is responsible for appetite and digestion; spleen qi deficiency produces poor appetite and loose stools. Lung qi is responsible for the strength of respiration; when it is deficient, a person experiences shortness of breath and a chronic cough. Treatment focuses on strengthening, or tonifying, the qi of the affected organs.

In disorders of sinking qi, the qi that holds organs in place has insufficient strength to do its job. The result is sagging, prolapsed organs, such as the uterus, transverse colon, or rectum. Specific acupuncture points and herbs can correct this type of imbalance.

When qi is stagnant, the functions of an organ are impaired due to a blockage in its qi flow. The liver is the organ most often affected by qi stagnation. Since the liver is in charge of the smooth flow of emotion, stagnant liver qi frequently results in irritability and anger. Because there is sufficient qi, tonifying in these cases would make the situation worse, so treatment focuses on moving qi away from the area.

In rebellious qi, the normal direction of organ qi is reversed. Each organ has a normal direction of qi flow; for example, the lungs and stomach move qi downward, while the spleen moves qi upward. Rebellious lung qi results in coughing or wheezing; rebellious stomach qi produces symptoms of nausea, belching, or vomiting; and rebellious spleen qi produces diarrhea.

BLOOD

In traditional Chinese medicine, blood has some parallels to its Western counterpart, such as its function of circulating through the body and nourishing the organs. However, it also has some very subtle functions in traditional Chinese medicine, such as providing a substantial foundation for the mind and improving sensitivity of the sensory organs. In other words, a deficiency of blood causes an impairment in mental function, leading to poor memory, anxiety, and insomnia. Blood deficiency can also impair the senses, especially the eyes, causing blurry vision. Closely aligned with qi, blood has a complementary relationship with it. The saying, "Blood is the mother of qi, and qi is the leader of blood," refers to the fact that without blood, qi has no fundamental nutritional basis; without qi, the body cannot form or circulate blood, and the blood would fail to stay within the vessels. The two are considered to flow together through the body.

DISORDERS OF BLOOD

Blood's main function is to circulate throughout the body, providing nourishment and moisture to the organs, skin, muscles, and tendons. When blood is deficient, symptoms such as dry skin and hair, inflexible tendons, and various emotional and reproductive imbalances can occur, depending on the organs involved. Since qi and blood are so closely related, a deficiency or stagnation of one of the substances often leads to the same type of imbalance in the other one.

Dry skin and hair are just two of the symptoms of a deficiency of blood.

The organs that have the most intimate relationship with blood are the spleen, heart, and liver. The spleen creates qi and blood from food; it also helps keep blood within the vessels. When spleen qi is deficient, blood deficiency or bleeding disorders can occur. The heart is said to "rule the blood and vessels." When it is qi or yang deficient, energy to move blood through the vessels is insufficient, resulting in poor circulation and feelings of coldness in the extremities. Since the heart blood is also the resting place for the mind and spirit, deficient heart blood leads to symptoms of insomnia, palpitations, restlessness, and poor memory. Finally, the liver stores the blood during times of rest or sleep. This function is a process of regeneration, and it is also intimately involved with menstrual flow and fertility. A deficiency of liver blood can lead to scanty menstruation or infertility. Stagnant liver blood may lead to menstrual cramping and discomfort. Since the liver opens into the eyes, this deficiency can also produce such symptoms as blurry vision, floaters, and dry eyes.

BODY FLUIDS

Body fluids refer to all the fluids in the body, such as sweat, tears, saliva, and various secretions and lubricants. The spleen and stomach regulate the formation of fluids, which are considered byproducts of digestion, while the intestines and bladder are involved in their excretion. The lungs regulate body fluids from above, and the kidneys are in charge of their metabolism throughout the body. Fluids consist of two basic types: clear thin fluids known as jin, and thick viscous fluids known as ye. Jin is distributed mostly to the muscles and skin, keeping them moist and nourished. Ye acts as a lubricant to the joints and nourishes the brain. Jin ye is the collective term for all the body fluids.

Because of the relationship between the organs and body fluids, a traditional Chinese medicine practitioner can extrapolate a wealth of information about organ function from the condition of the jin ye. For this reason, the initial interview includes questions about thirst, urination, color of fluids, and the amount and timing of sweating. Sweat is ruled by the heart. Excessive sweating during the day is considered a sign of yang deficiency; night sweats, on the other hand, are a sign of yin deficiency. Tears relate to the liver; dry eyes are a sign of liver blood and yin deficiency. Sputum is ruled by the spleen; excessive sputum is a symptom of yin excess in the spleen. The lungs are the storage area for mucus; a runny nose or wet cough is a sign of yin excess in the lungs. Since the kidneys control the moisture of the entire body, a dry mouth can indicate kidney yin deficiency.

The body fluids also have an intimate relationship with qi. Since qi is involved in the transformation of fluids, deficient qi can lead to fluid retention or excessive sweating. Conversely, fluid stagnation can impair qi circulation, and profuse loss of body fluid can lead to a severe deficiency of qi. For this reason, herbs that induce sweating are used cautiously in people who are qi deficient.

ESSENCE AND SPIRIT (JING AND SHEN)

Stored in the kidneys, essence (jing) is the subtle substance that is responsible for growth, development, and reproduction. Prenatal essence is inherited from the parents, and it is the original substance of life. It cannot be increased, but it can be conserved through a healthy lifestyle and moderation. It can be supplemented with postnatal essence, which is derived from nutrition. When the essence is strong, a child grows and develops normally and enjoys healthy brain function

Strong prenatal essence makes it possible for a child to grow and develop normally. When prenatal essence is deficient, mental retardation, birth defects, and an overall failure to thrive are possible.

and strong immunity and fertility as an adult. Conversely, birth defects, mental retardation, and a child's failure to thrive are considered signs of a deficiency of essence. In adults, essence deficiency can cause infertility, low immunity, and premature aging.

Spirit (shen) is a person's innate vitality. It can be considered the soul, but it also has a material aspect. When an individual has healthy shen, the eyes have the glow of life and the mind is clear. Since the heart is the resting place for the spirit, disturbances in shen are typically diagnosed as heart imbalances. A mild shen syndrome appears with a heart blood deficiency, with signs of forgetfulness, insomnia, fatigue, and restlessness. In a more serious shen syndrome, "heat phlegm confusing the heart," the individual may be violent, with red face and eyes; the Western diagnosis of this condition might be psychosis. A person who is in a coma as a result of a stroke or a person who experiences epileptic seizures may receive a diagnosis of the shen disturbance known as "phlegm blocking the heart opening."

CHAPTER 4:
The Internal Organs

The internal organs are responsible for the vital functions of the human body. The understanding and description of the internal organ structures and systems in traditional Chinese medicine is remarkably sophisticated, considering the fact that traditional organ theory was developed during Confucian times (approximately 559–479 B.C.). In this period, it was considered a violation of the sanctity of life to perform dissections, so the entire organ theory was developed on the basis of how the body functions. The body was viewed in a holistic sense, with the understanding that all functions necessary to maintain health were innately present within its internal organs. By means of careful observation, the Taoists were able to perceive functional relationships among seemingly unrelated activities, actions, emotions, and sensory perceptions.

The function and structure of the vital organs in traditional Chinese medicine differ from that of similarly named organs in Western medicine. It's true that in some cases, the functional relationships closely parallel those established in Western medicine. For example, the Taoists reasoned that "the kidneys govern water." Both traditional Chinese and Western medical systems recognize that the kidneys play an essential role in filtering and expelling waste water through the urinary bladder. But Chinese medical theory discusses the organs based not only on their function but on their relationship with other organs. In traditional organ theory, the kidneys are also responsible for reproduction and fertility; this theory has no counterpart in the Western anatomic concept of the organ. Yet, herbs that nourish "kidney essence" are quite effective clinically in promoting fertility.

It is important to let each medical system stand on its own rather than attempting to create a one-to-one correspondence between Western anatomy and the Taoist functional organ systems. Each system has its own strengths and weaknesses, and each is complete in its own way.

THE YIN ORGANS

In traditional Chinese medicine, the five yin organs, or solid (zang) organs, are the lungs, spleen, heart, liver, and kidneys. The pericardium is sometimes considered a sixth yin organ. The yin organs produce, transform, and store qi (see page 22), blood, body fluids, and essence.

THE LUNGS (FEI)

The lungs are considered the "tender organ" in Chinese medicine because they open directly to the external environment and are usually the first internal organ attacked by external pathogens (disease-causing organisms) such as bacteria or viruses. Symptoms of imbalance in the lungs include cough, asthma, phlegm, chest pain, bloating, loss of voice, and nosebleeds. The functions of the lungs in traditional Chinese medicine:

In traditional Chinese medicine, coughing is a sign that there is an imbalance in the lungs.

The lungs control breathing. This important function closely parallels the Western understanding of the organ. In addition to controlling inhalation of oxygen and exhalation of carbon dioxide, the lungs—along with the spleen—are seen as the source of postnatal qi, the actual vitality of a person. (The kidneys are considered the source of prenatal qi, the constitution.) The concept of postnatal qi is important because people with a weak constitution don't have to be consigned to a lifetime of fatigue or illness. Through breathing exercises such as qi gong, a person can enhance his or her vitality through the qi of the lungs.

The lungs control the qi of the entire body. Since the lungs transform inhaled air into qi, they have an important influence on the functional activities of the entire body. When lung qi is strong, breathing is normal and the body has sufficient energy. Weak lung qi, on the other hand, deprives the other organs and body tissues of energy, leading to shortness of breath, weak voice, and general fatigue.

The lungs control body fluids in the lower part of the body. An organ of the upper body, the lungs assist in moving qi and body fluids to the lower portion of the body. When this descending action of the lungs is impaired and normal qi flow is disrupted, cough and shortness of breath may occur. Also, fluids can collect in the upper body, resulting in edema (severe water retention) and difficulty in urination. If this concept is difficult to understand from a Western anatomic perspective, think of it from an energetic perspective. For example, when you dip a drinking straw into water, the straw fills with water. The water then flows out of the straw when you lift the straw out of the water. However, if you place a finger over the end of the straw before you lift it out of the water, the water remains in the straw until you lift your finger. This action is similar to the blockage of downward water movement that results from impairment in lung function.

The lungs govern body hair and skin. This principle refers to the lungs' function of dispersing moisture to the skin, maintaining its suppleness and elasticity. The body hair and pores are also considered an integral part of the lungs' defensive system: They act as the boundary between the outer environment and the interior of the body, protecting the body from the external environment. The qi that flows just under the skin is called wei qi and is considered the body's immune system.

Body hair and pores are considered part of the lungs' defensive system.

When the wei qi is strong, the body is able to fight off external pathogens. Clinically, the relationship between the lungs and the pores is seen in persons who frequently catch colds: They often complain that they have an aversion to wind, and they break into a sweat when they aren't feeling warm. These symptoms are due to an impairment of the lungs' control of the pores, resulting in the easy access to the body's interior by external pathogens.

The lungs open to the nose and control the voice. When lung qi is healthy, the sense of smell is acute, the nasal passages remain open, and the voice is strong. When lung qi experiences dysfunction, the person may experience symptoms of nasal congestion, excessive mucus, an impaired sense of smell, and a weak or hoarse voice. As most of us have experienced, a breakdown in energy throughout the body often follows these symptoms.

THE SPLEEN (PI)

Of all the organs in traditional Chinese medicine, the spleen bears the least resemblance to its Western counterpart. The latter deals primarily with production and destruction of red blood cells and storage of blood. In traditional Chinese physiology, the spleen plays a central part in the health and vitality of the body, taking a lead role in the assimilation of nutrients and maintenance of physical strength. It turns digested food from the stomach into usable nutrients and qi. Entire schools of medicine were formed around this organ; the premise was that all aspects of vitality depend on the entire body receiving proper nutrition from the healthy functioning of this essential organ.

Symptoms of imbalance in the spleen include a lack of appetite, muscular atrophy (wasting), indigestion, abdominal fullness, bloating, jaundice, and inappropriate bleeding or bruising. The traditional attributes possessed by the spleen:

The spleen governs transformation and transportation. Once the stomach breaks down and digests food, the spleen transforms it into usable nutrition and qi, then transports this food essence to the other organs. The spleen plays an essential role in the production of blood as well. For this reason, fatigue (qi deficiency) and anemia (blood deficiency) are often attributed to a breakdown in the spleen's ability to transform food into qi and blood. In addition to its role in nutrition and blood production, the spleen is also responsible for the "transformation of fluids": It assists in water metabolism, helping the body rid itself of excess fluid and moistening the areas that need it, such as the joints. If this function is disrupted, fluid disorders such as edema (severe water retention) or excessive phlegm can develop.

The spleen governs the blood. Considered the "foundation of postnatal existence," the spleen is the most important organ involved in the production of sufficient blood to maintain health. A highly nutritious diet appropriate to the individual's needs enhances the qi of the spleen, thus improving the person's energy level. These improvements are seen readily in clinical practice, where a sickly person can become quite strong through tonifying herbs, dietary changes, and breathing exercises. Spleen qi is also specifically responsible for keeping blood within the vessels. A weakness in this function can lead to chronic bleeding, such as a tendency to bruise easily, or breakthrough bleeding in the middle of the menstrual cycle.

The spleen dominates the muscles and four limbs. Since the spleen is responsible for transforming food into qi and blood and transporting them throughout the body, proper functioning of the organ is essential to maintain muscle mass and strong limbs. A person with deficient spleen qi often experiences weakness and fatigue in

While a healthy diet is good for the body, the spleen must be able to transmit this nutrition to the muscles for the body to benefit from it.

the limbs. Exercise and a healthy diet benefit the body only if the spleen is able to transmit this nutrition and energy to the muscles.

The spleen opens into the mouth and lips. As the gateway to the digestive system, the mouth can indicate whether the spleen is functioning normally. If qi is normal, appetite is good, the lips are red and supple, and the sense of taste is sufficiently sensitive.

Spleen qi moves in an upward direction. All organs have a normal direction for their flow of qi. The flow of spleen qi keeps other organs in their proper place. If spleen qi is weak, then prolapse, or sagging, of the transverse colon, uterus, rectum, or stomach can result.

The spleen likes warmth and dislikes cold. Since the digestive enzymes require warmth to break down food properly, excessive consumption of cold foods and drinks can impair spleen function. Foods that are warming and easy to digest, such as soups with grated ginger, benefit spleen function.

THE HEART (XIN)

Known in traditional Chinese physiology as the ruler of the other organs, the heart has exceptional importance. Its function in traditional Chinese medicine parallels its Western anatomic function of pumping blood throughout the body to maintain life, but in the Eastern tradition it is also intimately involved with mental and emotional processes. Considered the residence of the mind and spirit, the heart is the organ most often involved in psychological imbalances. Properly nourished and balanced, the heart maintains our innate wisdom, contentment, and emotional balance. Symptoms of heart imbalance include palpitations, shortness of breath, sweating easily, mental restlessness, insomnia, forgetfulness, chest pain, tongue pain, and burning urine. The traditional functions of the heart:

The heart controls the blood and blood vessels. When the heart is healthy, it pumps blood vigorously through the vessels to all parts of the body, nourishing the organs and maintaining vitality. A deficiency in this function can appear as pale complexion, cold hands and feet, palpitations, insomnia, and emotional disturbances.

The heart manifests on the face. When the heart is strong and possesses sufficient blood, the complexion is rosy, and the individual looks robust and healthy. When the heart blood is deficient, on the other hand, the person looks pale and unhealthy. If heart yang or qi is deficient, the complexion may appear bluish, especially in the lips.

The heart houses the shen (spirit) and mind. This function encompasses the full range of human consciousness, including emotional health, mental function, memory, and spirituality. When the yin of the heart is deficient, a person can experience symptoms such as palpitations, anxiety, insomnia, and restlessness. When the heart blood is deficient, poor memory, depression, and a tendency to be "spaced out" or "in the clouds" can result.

The heart opens onto the tongue. In Chinese physiology, when an internal organ opens onto a sensory organ, it means the two organs are linked through structure, function, or physiology. By examining the sensory organ, a practitioner can determine much about the health of the internal organ linked to it. The tongue (the organ of taste) can indicate health or imbalance in all the organs. A pale tongue can indicate heart blood deficiency, while a red tongue with no coating may indicate heart yin deficiency. On another level, "the heart controls speech." Heart deficiency syndromes can lead to a withdrawn, quiet demeanor, for example. One patient who sought acupuncture treatment had experienced a complete loss of voice after a traumatic experience. While receiving strong acupuncture stimulation in a heart channel point on the wrist, the patient got angry and shouted, "Do you realize how much that hurts?" After apologizing to the patient for the unexpected discomfort, the practitioner reminded him that he had just spoken for the first time in a week! This sort of dramatic release of emotional trauma is quite common in acupuncture therapy, and it usually leads to a feeling of well-being afterward, as it did in this case.

The Liver (Gan)

The liver plays an important role in traditional Chinese physiology. Since it is in charge of the smooth flow of qi throughout the body, any disruption in its functions usually affects another organ. Stagnation of the flow of liver qi frequently disrupts emotional flow, producing feelings of frustration or anger. Conversely, these same emotions can lead to a dysfunction in the liver, resulting in an endless loop of cause and effect.

Anger and frustration can result from stagnation of the flow of liver qi. These emotions, in turn, can lead to liver dysfunction.

Associated with the storage of blood, the liver is also the primary organ involved in a woman's menstrual cycle. When the liver is out of balance, the following symptoms can occur: emotional problems, rib pain or fullness, dizziness, headache, cramping, tendon problems, menstrual problems, jaundice, weak or blurry vision, and digestive disorders. The functions of the liver:

The liver stores the blood. The liver is considered a storage area for blood when blood is not being used for physical activity. These periods of rest contribute to the body's restorative processes. During exercise, the blood is released to nourish the tendons and muscles. This function is also intimately associated with the menstrual cycle; the liver maintains an adequate blood supply and regulates the timing and comfort of menstruation. Any dysfunctions in the menstrual cycle are almost always treated through the regulation of liver blood, qi, or yin. When liver qi is stagnant (a very common condition), a person experiences irritability, tightness in the chest, and, in a woman, symptoms of premenstrual syndrome. When liver blood is deficient, symptoms such as dry eyes and skin, pallor, and lack of menstruation can occur.

The liver ensures the smooth flow of qi. The *Nei Jing* refers to the liver as a general in the army, coordinating the movement of the troops. When the liver functions smoothly, physical and emotional activity throughout the body also runs smoothly. When the liver's ability to spread qi smoothly throughout the body is disrupted due to stress or lifestyle choices, however, the liver qi can become either stagnant or hyperactive, causing havoc in other organs, such as the lungs, stomach, and spleen. Often, stress-related problems such as irritable bowel syndrome or indigestion can be successfully treated by working through the "smoothing of liver qi."

The liver controls the tendons. As discussed previously, the liver stores blood during periods of rest and then releases it to the muscles and tendons in times of activity. When liver blood is deficient, tightness and inflexibility in the muscles and tendons can result. If liver qi is stagnant, muscles can go into spasm. Such muscle spasms often occur when a person drinks strong coffee. Coffee, even the decaffeinated variety, is one of the most disruptive substances in relation to the smooth flow of liver qi. Many people experience a tightness in the shoulder muscles and neck muscles after ingesting this powerful herbal stimulant. In fact, it can be extremely difficult to resolve liver imbalances in people who drink coffee regularly.

The liver opens into the eyes. Although all the organs have some connection to the health of the eyes, the liver is connected to proper eye function. Chronic eye problems can usually be traced to a deficiency of liver yin or blood, for example. It is quite common to resolve eye disorders successfully by treating the liver.

The liver shows on the nails. When liver blood is plentiful, it spreads to the farthest areas of the body, including the fingernails and toenails. When liver blood is deficient, on the other hand, the nails can appear pale, weak, and brittle.

THE KIDNEYS (SHEN)

Although the kidneys' function of regulating water metabolism in Chinese physiology closely parallels their function in Western medicine, their influence is much more far-reaching. They are the storage place for vital essence (jing), a subtle substance responsible for growth, development, reproduction, and fertility. They are also considered the source of yin and yang for all the other organs, so a chronic disruption in their function can potentially affect any other part of the body. The kidneys are the source of prenatal qi, which is inherited from the parents and interpreted as a person's innate constitution. Ultimately, the health and strength of the kidneys is the major determining factor in a person's long-term vitality and longevity. Symptoms of imbalance in the kidneys include low back pain, infertility, impotence or excessive sexual desire, urinary problems, tinnitus or deafness, edema, or asthma. The traditional functions of the kidneys:

The kidneys store essence (jing). Jing, or essence, is a subtle substance that underlies all organic life processes. While it includes reproductive fluids, its scope goes far beyond this one area. There are two main types of essence: prenatal and postnatal. Prenatal essence is derived from the genetic material of the parents as well as the vitality of their lifestyle, habits, and nutrition. It is essentially a person's inherited constitution at birth. Postnatal essence, on the other hand, is within a person's control because it is derived from food and air. It is possible for a person who has a weak prenatal essence to lead a vital and healthy life through the maintenance of a strong postnatal essence. A healthy diet and lifestyle, along with exercise and breathing practices, such as qi gong, are the means to achieving strong postnatal essence. (See page 146 for more on qi gong.) In fact, a person with a weak constitution and a healthy lifestyle is better off than a person with a strong constitution and an unhealthy lifestyle. The latter often goes for years without any illness and then suddenly succumbs to cancer or heart disease. The person with weaker prenatal essence, on the other hand, is unable to get away with an unhealthy lifestyle because he or she gets immediate feedback in the form of illness or fatigue.

Even if a person is born with weak prenatal essence, they can lead a healthy, vital life by strengthening their postnatal qi through healthy eating, regular exercise, and breathing practices such as qi gong.

The kidneys control water metabolism. The balance of yin and yang in the kidneys determines the efficiency of water metabolism in the body. When kidney yang or kidney qi are deficient, excessive urination or edema (swelling due to severe fluid retention) may occur.

The kidneys grasp the qi. While the lungs are the body's major organ of respiration, the kidneys provide the "grasping" force that is necessary for full inhalation. When kidney yang or kidney qi is deficient, therefore, a person may suffer a difficulty in inhalation, as is experienced by people with asthma.

The kidneys control the bones. According to Chinese physiology, the kidneys are also responsible for the development of strong bones. When the kidneys are deficient, a person may have brittle bones and, subsequently, repeated injuries and poor dental health.

The kidneys produce marrow and are connected to the brain. Marrow has a much broader function in traditional Chinese medicine than it has in Western medicine. In the latter, it is involved primarily in bone and blood-cell growth. In Chinese physiology, marrow is derived directly from essence, and it is the source of the substance that makes up the brain. Deficiencies in essence or marrow can appear in cases of mental retardation.

The kidneys open into the ear. This function has great clinical significance: Hearing difficulties can often be treated by nourishing the kidneys. Babies are considered to have undeveloped hearing capacity due to the lack of maturation of kidney energy; elderly people tend to have ringing in the ears (tinnitus) or impaired hearing due to a depletion of their kidney qi over time.

THE PERICARDIUM (XIN BAO)

The pericardium provides a shield around the heart to protect it against external pathogenic factors. Sometimes considered a sixth yin organ, it has no separate functions of its own.

The six yang organs, or hollow (fu) organs, are generally considered to be less significant in their functions than are the yin organs. The yang organs serve primarily to separate impure substances from food and then drain them out of the body as waste material. Each yang organ is paired with a yin organ. For example, the spleen and the stomach together encompass the digestive process. The stomach performs the yang function of processing the food and passing it on; the spleen performs the yin function of extracting nourishment from the food and transforming it into qi and blood. The following are the functions of the stomach and the other five yang organs: the small intestine, large intestine, urinary bladder, gallbladder, and "triple burner."

THE STOMACH (WEI)

As explained above, the stomach is paired with the spleen. It is the beginning of the digestive process, and its functions act as a yang complement to the spleen's yin functions. Symptoms of stomach dysfunction include excessive or impaired appetite, nausea, vomiting, excessive or insufficient thirst, and mouth sores. Its normal functions in traditional Chinese medicine:

The stomach is responsible for receiving and ripening food. The stomach functions as a cauldron in "rotting and ripening" food to prepare it for the spleen's extraction of its essence. Considered the "middle burner" when paired with the spleen, its proper functioning is essential for health and vitality.

The stomach controls digestion of food and water. If the stomach is weak in its ability to prepare food for digestion, the spleen is unable to create sufficient qi and blood, resulting in weakness or impairment in other organs. The stomach also begins the process of "separating the pure from the impure." It sends the pure essence of food and fluids onward to the next yin organ for storage and transformation; the impure waste is sent to the next yang organ to be further processed or eliminated from the body.

Stomach qi moves downward. When the stomach qi functions properly, it has a downward movement. After the stomach separates the pure essence and transfers it to the spleen, the "rotted and ripened" (digested) food is sent downward to the small intestine for further processing. If this downward energy is disrupted, however, the stomach qi moves upward. Known as rebellious stomach qi, this upward movement produces symptoms of nausea, vomiting, belching, hiccups, and acid regurgitation (often called acid reflux in the West).

The stomach likes dampness and dislikes dryness. Since the stomach is a yang organ, it tends to overheat when it is out of balance. Maintaining a moist atmosphere with sufficient fluids in the stomach helps to ward off stomach yin deficiency. This can be achieved by avoiding alcohol, excessive spices, and dry foods (such as popcorn, bread, crackers, and dried fruit) that are consumed without fluids.

The use of excessive spices in the diet can lead to a deficiency of fluids in the stomach, which in turn can result in a deficiency in stomach yin.

Small Intestine (Xiao Chang)

The small intestine is paired with the heart in a yin/yang relationship. Symptoms of imbalance in the small intestine are lower abdominal pain, bloating, indigestion, gas, diarrhea, dark, burning urine, or blood in the urine. The functions of the small intestine are:

The small intestine separates the clear and dirty aspects of food and produces urine. After the stomach sends the pure essence of food to the spleen, it sends the rest of the food to the small intestine, where further processing takes place. The spleen once again receives the "clear" aspect of the digested food (the nutrients), while the "dirty" part (the waste) is sent down to the large intestine. After food has been further processed, any impure fluids remaining are sent to the kidneys and bladder, where they are excreted as urine.

Large Intestine (Da Chang)

The large intestine continues the process of digestion: It receives waste, absorbs fluids, and excretes feces. It is paired with the lungs. Disorders of the large intestine can lead to constipation, diarrhea, or lower abdominal pain. Its traditional functions:

The large intestine passes dirty qi and waste out of the body. After receiving the turbid material from the small intestine, the large intestine is the final stage of processing digested food. The final waste products of digestion are formed into stools and passed from the body.

The large intestine controls body fluids. As the final stage of fluid metabolism, the large intestine absorbs water from the products of digestion while forming stools. A disruption in this function can lead to diarrhea (too much fluid) or constipation (insufficient fluid).

Chinese Healing Secrets

Urinary Bladder (Pang Guang)

The urinary bladder's role is the same as it is in the West, storing urine and discharging it periodically. It is paired with the kidneys. Symptoms of bladder dysfunction include difficulty urinating, with burning, pain, urgency, bleeding, and retention. The traditional function of the urinary bladder:

The urinary bladder receives and excretes urine. After receiving turbid fluids from the lungs, small intestine, and large intestine, the kidneys extract the last of the pure essence. The turbid remnants are then sent to the bladder, where they are stored until they are excreted from the body through urination.

Gallbladder (Dan)

The gallbladder is paired with the liver; liver disharmonies often affect the gallbladder and vice versa. Disharmonies of the gallbladder can produce symptoms such as intercostal pain (pain between the ribs), anger, rash decisions, timidity, digestive problems, and emotional disturbances. Normal gallbladder functions:

The gallbladder stores and secretes bile. The liver produces bile and the gallbladder stores it. When you eat fatty foods, the gallbladder contracts and pours bile into the small intestine to assist in digestion. Over-consumption of fatty foods can adversely affect the function of the liver and gallbladder.

The gallbladder rules decisions. An indecisive, timid person is said to have a weak gallbladder. A person who acts impulsively or out of anger, on the other hand, could be suffering from an excess yang condition in the gallbladder.

Chinese Healing Secrets

TRIPLE BURNER (SAN JIAO)

The triple burner is not an organ per se, but rather it is a grouping of organs by function and location. The triple burner is paired with the pericardium in a yin/yang relationship. The primary function of the triple burner organs is water metabolism, and the organs are grouped as follows:

Upper Burner: Comprising the heart and lungs, the upper burner is described as a "fog" or "mist." It disperses the essence of food and qi throughout the body. Illness usually attacks this burner first, then it proceeds to the middle and lower burners.

Middle Burner: The spleen and stomach function together as the middle burner, acting as a "foam." Metabolism in this burner involves churning food and water into a digestible, souplike consistency. Digestive disorders are often described as middle burner imbalances.

Lower Burner: The lower burner encompasses the organs below the navel: the intestines, kidneys, and bladder. It is considered a "swamp," since it is the sewage system of the body, excreting waste.

THE EXTRA OR "CURIOUS" ORGANS

The curious organs are so named because their existence can be confirmed through observation, but they don't fall into any particular category. They are the marrow, bones, blood vessels, brain, uterus, and gallbladder. Although the gallbladder is classified as a yang organ, it is also considered a curious organ since it is the only yang organ that stores a vital substance (bile). The marrow is a vital essence stored by the kidneys. It is related to growth and development and nourishes the brain. The functions of the other organs parallel their Western counterparts.

Chinese Healing Secrets

CHAPTER 5:
Patterns of Disharmony

Over the centuries, a sophisticated system of diagnosis has evolved in traditional Chinese medicine. By following various established diagnostic procedures, a practitioner of traditional Chinese medicine can construct a detailed picture of the status of all the internal organs without the aid of laboratory tests or other types of modern technology. To identify a pattern of disharmony, the physician will assess the status of the organs, gradually uncovering the cause of the disease by grouping the symptoms into traditional patterns.

TRADITIONAL PATTERNS OF DISHARMONY

During the initial patient visit, the practitioner must organize all of the seemingly unrelated facts gathered about a patient's condition, gradually refining this information into diagnostic categories. At first, the practitioner organizes the evidence loosely into general categories known as the eight parameters, which consist of four groups of polarities: yin and yang, heat and cold, internal and external, excess and deficiency. This eight-parameter diagnosis is the basic foundation for all diagnostic categories. It gives the practitioner a general overview of the patient's disease, or pattern of disharmony. Once the practitioner has grouped

Through various diagnostic procedures, the traditional Chinese medicine practitioner evaluates the status of the internal organs.

the symptoms according to the eight parameters, he or she can further refine the diagnosis to determine the condition of the vital substances and internal organs. In this way, the diagnosis evolves from a general image into a specific, clear description of the individual patient's physiologic processes. For example, in organ diagnosis, spleen qi deficiency is a pattern of disharmony. This is a very specific diagnosis. In eight-parameter diagnosis, the same imbalance is classified generally as a deficient internal condition.

THE EIGHT PARAMETERS

It's important to remember that in traditional Chinese medicine, illness is seen as an imbalance, a lack of harmony in the body's systems. This disharmony is understood in terms of the eight principal parameters. Knowledge of the eight parameters allows the practitioner to perceive the location, severity, and nature of the disease process. This information is then applied to the other diagnostic categories of qi, blood, and internal organs, further narrowing and focusing the diagnosis. It is also important to remember that a physical condition is not fixed; inner processes are always subject to change. In other words, a yin condition can evolve into a yang condition; an exterior pattern can penetrate to the interior; a cold condition might turn to heat; and an excess disease often becomes one of deficiency. In a more complex disharmony, all eight patterns could occur simultaneously! For this reason, it is always a good idea to maintain a Taoist attitude of flexibility while perceiving the movements of nature. Any diagnostic pattern is simply a snapshot in time; an experienced practitioner recognizes this and is always prepared to adjust the diagnosis and treatment plan to accommodate these changes.

Chinese Healing Secrets

External / Internal:

The terms external (or exterior) and internal (or interior) do not refer to where the pathogen comes from; rather, they specify the location of the disease process in the body. The exterior of the body is considered the skin and muscles, while the interior is defined as the internal organs and bones. In an external pattern, the pathogen fights with the body's defensive qi, or wei qi, which circulates under the skin. Symptoms of this struggle are chills, fever, sensitivity to wind or cold, body aches, sore throat, nasal congestion, and a floating pulse. (The different pulses and their role in diagnosis are explained on pages 124–126.) If the cause of disease, known in traditional Chinese medicine as the pernicious influence (see pages 58–72), is not expelled, typically it penetrates the interior. An interior, or internal, condition has more organ-related symptoms, such as diarrhea, stomachache, intestinal cramps, lung pain, bladder pain, constipation, and changes in the color of the tongue. A pathogen trapped between the interior and exterior exhibits such symptoms as alternating chills and fever, a bitter taste in the mouth, and a wiry pulse.

Heat / Cold:

The possible causes of heat conditions are an external heat pernicious influence (for example, a virus that produces heat symptoms, such as a high fever), internal hyperactivity of yang functions (for example, drinking too much alcohol can cause a red face and headache), or insufficient yin. The yin aspect of the body includes the "lubricating and cooling" systems. When these systems are depleted,

Drinking too much alcohol can cause a heat condition.

the body tends to overheat due to the deficiency of yin. In general, heat signs include redness in the face; feeling hot; thirst; colored secretions (such as yellow mucus or other discharges or dark urine); constipation; burning sensations; irritability; red tongue body with a yellow coating; and a rapid pulse.

Conversely, cold arises from external cold pernicious influences (for example, a virus that produces the cold symptoms of chills and a runny nose), an internal yang deficiency, or internal excess cold pathogenic factors. An internal yang deficiency produces such symptoms as always feeling cold, a low sex drive, and low energy. A person who has acute symptoms of loose stools and abdominal pains from eating too much ice cream likely has an internal excess cold condition. General signs of cold are a pale face, feelings of cold, lack of thirst, clear secretions (pale urine, clear mucus or discharges), loose stools, muscle tightness, fatigue, pale tongue with a white coating, and a slow pulse.

EXCESS / DEFICIENCY

A disease is classified as an excess condition or a deficient condition. Excess conditions occur when an external pernicious influence attacks the body and creates overactivity (for example, a high fever that is caused by infection with a virus); a body function becomes overactive (for example, redness and swelling that are caused by an infection); or an obstruction of qi or blood causes pain. Acute conditions tend to be conditions of excess.

Deficient conditions arise due to an inherent weakness in the body or a weakness in the body's vital energy (qi), blood, yin, or yang. Symptoms of deficiency include weak movement, pale face, pale tongue, and weak pulse. Chronic conditions tend to be conditions of deficiency.

The most general of all the diagnostic categories, it can be considered a summary of all the others. Heat, excess, and external conditions are yang conditions, while cold, deficiency, and internal conditions are yin conditions. Most conditions include a mixture of yin and yang imbalances. In addition, each internal organ has its yin and yang aspects that must be balanced. For example, if heart yin is deficient, a person may experience insomnia, poor memory, and palpitations. If heart yang is depleted, poor circulation, pale face, purple lips, edema, and cold extremities can result. When yin, with its cooling function, is low, heat signs occur. When yang, with its heating function, is low, cold signs occur. Restoring the optimum yin/yang balance of each internal organ is the most important secret of maintaining health and vitality in traditional Chinese medicine.

SYNDROMES OF QI, BLOOD, YIN, AND YANG

Analyzing disease according to the eight parameters is essential in arriving at a diagnosis. However, it is only the first step; it usually does not provide enough information for a truly focused treatment plan. For example, a person might have chronic fatigue—according to the eight parameters, chronic fatigue indicates an internal deficiency. The practitioner might recognize at this point that the person needs tonifying herbs to nourish and alleviate the deficiency, but which herbs? With further inquiry, the practitioner learns that the person also has loose stools and a poor appetite. Since these symptoms are related to the functions of spleen qi, the practitioner now knows that the syndrome is an internal deficiency of spleen qi. By combining the eight parameters with knowledge of the vital substances and the organs, the diagnosis is now detailed enough to make a focused treatment plan: Tonify spleen qi. Tonifying herbs improve overall function of a particular organ and strengthen the entire organism when used long term.

Remember that qi flows in a system of channels, called meridians, in the body, and each organ is linked to a meridian. Acupuncture can affect or manipulate qi to treat a specific imbalance. A practitioner might choose herbs that tonify spleen qi and use acupuncture or moxibustion (the application of heat) at acupuncture points that affect the spleen. For example, a point on the spleen meridian known as Spleen 6 can be activated to strengthen the spleen. Since the spleen and stomach meridians are directly connected, needling or applying moxibustion to a point on the stomach meridian (Stomach 36) also strengthens the spleen. In this way, a wide variety of treatment options are available to a practitioner once an accurate diagnosis is at hand. See the chapter "Treatments in Traditional Chinese Medicine" for a discussion of various treatment options.

By stimulating specific points along the meridians through acupuncture, the practitioner can affect or manipulate the patient's qi. This manipulation can be used alone or with other therapies, such as herbal prescriptions, to treat specific imbalances.

DISORDERS OF QI

There are four disorders of qi: deficient qi, stagnant qi, sinking qi, and rebellious qi. When qi is deficient, the principal symptoms are fatigue, a bright pale face, a weak or soft voice, spontaneous sweating, a pale tongue, and a weak pulse. These general symptoms could occur in any type of qi deficiency. A further delineation of symptoms based on the organ system affected by the deficiency is described later (see Chapter 6). The treatment is to tonify qi.

Another type of qi imbalance is stagnant qi, an excess type of disharmony. Since health depends on the smooth flow of qi, stagnant qi can cause discomfort or pain almost anywhere in the body. It is typically associated with feelings of pain or distention that move from place to place, irritability, and soft lumps anywhere on the body that come and go. Premenstrual syndrome is a condition of stagnant qi in the liver. The treatment principle is to smooth the flow of qi through the affected organs or meridians.

In the disorder of sinking qi, a deficiency syndrome, the function of supporting the organs is impaired. Prolapse (sagging) of the bladder, rectum, transverse colon, or uterus occurs. Herbs that have an uplifting action, along with acupuncture and moxibustion, are used to treat this condition (see Chapter 8, "Treatments in Traditional Chinese Medicine," for more on acupuncture and moxibustion).

Finally, in patterns of rebellious qi, the flow of qi is the reverse of normal. For example, the normal direction of flow for stomach qi is downward. When rebellious stomach qi occurs, symptoms of nausea, vomiting, belching, or hiccups exist. The treatment principle is to return the flow of qi to normal, usually with herbs and acupuncture treatments. It is also necessary to rectify any underlying excess or deficiency that caused the problem.

DISORDERS OF BLOOD

Three types of blood disorders can occur: deficiency, stagnation, and excess of heat. Blood deficiency syndrome is especially common among women due to their monthly loss of menstrual blood. It can also arise as a result of improper nutrition or spleen qi deficiency, which prevents full assimilation of nutrients. Symptoms include a dull pale face, pale lips, pale tongue, dizziness, blurry vision, numbness or tingling of extremities, poor memory, dry skin and hair, scanty menses, and a thin pulse. The treatment principle is to tonify the blood with herbs, acupuncture, or moxibustion.

In blood stagnation, which is an excess pattern, the primary symptom is a fixed, stabbing pain, which can occur anywhere in the body as a result of injury, stagnation of qi or cold, or deficient blood conditions. Tumors or painful menstrual flow with clots may also occur. The treatment depends on the nature of the stagnation, but the common treatment principle is to activate or move the blood with herbs that stimulate circulation. Acupuncture is especially effective in treating the pain resulting from the stagnation.

With an excess condition of heat in the blood, symptoms of hemorrhage, skin rashes, itchiness, blood mixed in with bodily secretions, irritability, and sensations of heat can occur. Treatment includes using herbs that cool the blood along with hemostatic herbs to stop the bleeding.

Examination of the patient's tongue can tell the practitioner much about the type of imbalance affecting the patient.

DISORDERS OF YIN

In disorders of yin deficiency, the cooling, moistening action of the body is depleted, leading to symptoms of reddish cheeks, red tongue with little or no coat, dry throat, heat in the "five palms" (palms, soles, and sternum; sometimes called "five hearts"), night sweats, irritability, and a small, rapid pulse. The presence of additional symptoms depends on the organ system affected. The treatment principle is to tonify the yin and clear deficiency heat. In conditions of yin excess, there can be feelings of cold, mucus, and a general sluggishness. Treatment varies, depending on the particular type of excess yin, but it usually involves the use of warming herbs or diuretics.

DISORDERS OF YANG

Yang deficiency is a chronic syndrome characterized by cold extremities, lack of sexual desire, infertility, an aversion to cold, pale face, tongue, and lips, and a slow, weak pulse. Other signs and symptoms depend on the particular organ systems affected. The treatment principle is to tonify the yang. In yang excess disorders, signs and symptoms include headache, body aches, fever, sweating, thirst, red eyes, concentrated urine, constipation, mental restlessness, a red tongue with a yellow coating, and a full, rapid pulse. In this condition, the treatment principle is to clear excess heat.

THE CAUSES OF DISHARMONY

Practitioners of traditional Chinese medicine consider a number of factors in determining the cause of illness. Some of these causes are considered external, as in the six pernicious influences: wind, cold, heat, dryness, dampness, and summer heat. Other causes are considered internal, as in the seven emotions: anger, joy, worry, pensiveness, sadness, fear, and shock. Other factors that play a role in the development of disease are diet, lifestyle, and accidents. When the body is healthy, its various substances and energies are in harmonious balance, both internally and in relation to the external environment. When this innate vitality (true qi) and immune defenses (wei qi) are strong, it is difficult for externally contracted disease to gain a foothold, especially if the invading pathogen is weak. However, an exceptionally strong pathogen can overwhelm even a healthy person, especially if the person has been weakened by stress, fatigue, overwork, or other lifestyle factors. For example, a person with a strong immune system might avoid catching a cold, even if a sick person sneezes on him. However, if he

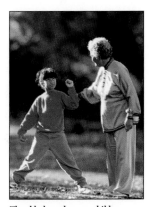

drinks a test tube full of the same virus, his strong immune system will be no match for such an onslaught. On the other hand, a person with very weak wei qi can catch whatever pathogen may be around due to his or her exceptionally weak defenses. This is the reason the elderly and young children are most at risk during influenza epidemics. This interplay between wei qi (also called good qi) and pathogenic factors (evil qi) determines whether a person gets sick, how the body responds to illness, and how long it takes for health to return.

The elderly and young children are the most at risk during influenza epidemics because their immune defenses, known as wei qi, tend to be weaker.

THE SIX PERNICIOUS INFLUENCES

Also known as the six pathogenic factors, six excesses, or six evils, these are the causes of disease that often arise from outside the body. They are wind, cold, heat, dampness, dryness, and summer heat. Although Western medicine recognizes only viruses and bacteria as

Chinese Healing Secrets

external pathogens, the Chinese observed that the body mirrors certain climatic conditions. (This follows the Taoist principle that "the macrocosm is within the microcosm" as described on page 19.) Although a diagnosis of "wind and cold invading the lungs" might sound primitive, this type of diagnosis accurately describes the way a certain type of pathogenic factor behaves inside the human body. The wind symptoms act just like wind in nature: They come and go, often without warning. Similarly, the cold symptoms act as they do in nature: They cause contraction, they slow functions down, and they make the person feel cold.

The high degree of effectiveness in treating this type of disorder (such as with herbs that "repel wind and scatter cold") is proof that the diagnosis is much more than a mere philosophical idea. Although Western medicine might be able to isolate the virus causing this condition, it still has no safe and effective way of treating the virus, other than relieving some of the symptoms it causes. On the other hand, thousands of years of trial and error through observation of nature and the human body have led to numerous effective treatments in Chinese medicine for viral infections that fit this pattern.

When learning about and discussing the various internal "climates" of the human body, it is important to remember that they may not always match the external climate. It is quite common for a person to develop symptoms of cold and dampness in rainy winter weather, but it is also possible to develop heat symptoms under the same weather conditions. Illness is the combination of the particular pathogen involved and a person's unique response to it. It is also possible for the pernicious influences to arise from internal causes. In this case, they usually result from a chronic internal imbalance. Descriptions of the six pernicious influences follow.

WIND

The pernicious influence of wind is considered the major cause of illness in traditional Chinese patterns of disharmony. It combines readily with other pathogens, giving rise to syndromes known as wind cold, wind heat, and wind dampness. This pathogenic factor possesses the qualities of wind in nature, appearing without warning and constantly changing. Considered a yang form of evil qi (a pathogenic factor), it often attacks the upper body, head, throat, and eyes. Wind causes movement, so it is usually involved when there are symptoms of twitching, spasms, or shaking. The organ most often affected by external wind is the lung; internal wind most commonly is related to an imbalance in the liver.

Syndromes of Wind

Wind Cold: In this syndrome, the pernicious influence of wind combines with that of cold. The person experiences symptoms of chills, fever (which is less severe than the chills), no sweating, headache, nasal congestion, and stiffness and pain in the shoulders, upper back, neck, and occipital area (back of the head). Cold causes objects to contract, and its effects in the body are no different. It causes chills, and the shivering causes the muscles to become tight and stiff. Although actual shivering may not occur, the person has difficulty staying warm, even when dressed properly for the conditions. Wind cold is traditionally treated with warm, diaphoretic (sweat-inducing) herbs to disperse the cold and repel the wind.

Wind Heat: Caused by a combination of pathogens, this syndrome is seen typically in the common cold or flu. The person may have symptoms of red face, high fever, sore throat, red eyes, thirst, red tongue, and a rapid pulse. Treatment for wind heat syndrome includes herbs that clear heat and repel wind.

Wind Damp: Arthritis is a manifestation of this pattern. Like dampness in nature, which is persistent and requires time to eradicate, the dampness pathogenic influence is difficult to cure and takes some time to resolve. The influence of wind also causes the pain to migrate from joint to joint, sometimes disappearing for a while only to reappear without warning. Treatment for this syndrome includes herbs that drain dampness and improve circulation of qi and blood through the affected areas. Moxibustion therapy—the application of heat—is particularly helpful in this situation.

Wind Water: This is a sudden attack of edema (swelling due to severe fluid retention), usually from allergies, poisoning, or acute nephritis (inflammation of the kidney). Diaphoretic (sweat-inducing) or diuretic (urine-producing) herbs are used along with acupuncture and moxibustion to treat this condition. The herbs help the body eliminate fluid, moxibustion helps the body metabolize fluids and improves circulation, and acupuncture moves stagnant fluids and expels the pathogenic factor.

Wind Rash: This category includes any skin condition that appears suddenly. Since dampness often plays a role in this condition, it can be difficult to treat. Treatment can include herbs that "scatter wind, clear heat, and drain dampness." For example, if the rash is red and burns, herbs that clear heat are

Because it heats the blood and increases wind, coffee should be avoided in skin conditions.

also used. Monitoring the diet is always an essential part of treatment. Coffee, in particular, should be avoided in skin conditions, since it heats up the blood, further increasing the wind.

Liver Wind Moving Internally: This is an internal condition of the liver that can result from a long-term imbalance; the usual chronic patterns are liver yin deficiency or blood deficiency. Signs of this condition are various abnormal body movements, such as twitching, shaking, convulsions, and spasms. The liver is in charge of the smooth movement of qi and blood in the body as well as harmonious movement within the body. An imbalance in the liver impairs this function, producing abnormal movement, and the influence of wind stirs this movement at unpredictable times.

Excessive Heat Producing Wind: If heat is too extreme, it can cause a sudden collapse, as in heatstroke. It can also cause sudden convulsions, such as those that occur in children with a high fever. Compare this internal process with what happens in nature when rising hot air causes gusts of high wind.

Blood Deficiency Leading to Wind: Since the liver stores blood, a deficiency of blood affects the liver, leading to wind. This condition can produce numbness and cramping. When the blood is tonified, these symptoms disappear.

COLD

The cold pathogenic factor is considered a yin evil qi. Its nature is to slow movement down, causing tightness, contraction, stagnation, and impaired circulation. When it is an external pathogenic factor, cold can attack the skin, muscles, and lungs. When it is an internal pathogenic factor, cold can cause an impairment in the normal functions of the spleen, stomach, and kidneys.

Syndromes of Cold

Wind Cold: In combination with the pathogenic factor of wind, cold attacks the exterior of the body and the lungs, causing chills, lack of sweating, occipital headache (pain at the base of the skull), upper body aches, tight shoulders and neck, and a congested nose. The influence of wind causes the symptoms to appear suddenly and affect the upper body, while cold causes the muscles to contract, causing the stiffness and pain. Nasal secretions are clear—another sign of cold. The treatment principle is to repel the wind and disperse the cold with warm diaphoretic herbs, acupuncture, and moxibustion.

Obstruction Due to Cold: Traditionally known as cold bi (blockage) pain, this condition typically takes the form of body aches or joint pain that is relieved by warmth. The most common Western diagnosis for this pattern is arthritis. Since the syndrome is caused by cold, the joint may actually feel cold to the touch, and the pain typically gets worse in cold weather. The Chinese treatment principle is to increase circulation and warm the acupuncture meridians through which qi and blood circulate by means of moxibustion, acupuncture, and herbs.

Cold Attacking the Spleen and Stomach: In this externally caused disorder, cold causes digestive symptoms such as abdominal pain, clear vomit, and watery diarrhea. Although it usually accompanies an externally contracted cold or stomach bacteria or virus (what we commonly refer to as stomach "flu"), this syndrome can also be caused by eating cold foods such as ice cream.

Chinese Healing Secrets

Cold Congealing the Liver Meridian: The liver meridian passes through the genital area, and this condition is a manifestation of cold in that meridian. Symptoms include testicular pain or shrinking and hernia pain. Moxibustion, acupuncture, and herbs can effectively correct this imbalance in a short time.

Spleen Yang Deficiency: If a person has an underlying deficiency of spleen yang (deficiency in energy and heat needed in order to digest food), cold can severely impair digestive function. Symptoms of spleen yang deficiency include watery stools with undigested food, cold extremities, edema, and a slow pulse. When a person with this underlying deficiency is also affected by external cold pathogens, the imbalance is especially difficult to eliminate. Treatment first expels the cold pathogenic factor. Then it tonifies the yang aspect of the spleen and kidneys to bring about a long-term increase in the body's basic metabolism, or its ability to maintain the heat needed for proper digestion, which is known in traditional Chinese medicine as life-gate (metabolic) fire. Spleen yang deficiency is treated with moxibustion and warming herbs that tonify spleen yang. This syndrome is discussed in greater detail in the section "Disorders of the Internal Organs" (page 83).

Kidney Yang Deficiency: Since the kidneys are the source of yang metabolic fire for the entire body, a deficiency in kidney yang can make the individual especially prone to cold. The symptoms of kidney yang deficiency include an inability to stay warm, cold extremities, low sex drive, frequent urination, edema (fluid retention), and pain in the low back. The yang deficiency can be corrected with long-term application of moxibustion and consumption of herbs that tonify kidney yang, thereby increasing metabolic fire.

Heat, or fire, is a yang pernicious influence that, when out of balance, can cause irritability, fever, and inflammation.

Heat, or fire, is a yang pernicious influence. As in nature, heat causes expansion and increased activity. When out of balance, heat can lead to irritability, fever, and inflammatory conditions. By its nature, heat rises, appearing as a red face and eyes, sore throat, and dizziness. If heat affects the heart or liver, anger may result. Heat tends to affect the body fluids, leading to thirst, constipation, and dark urine. Since it can produce wind, heat can lead to spasms.

Syndromes of Heat

Wind Heat: This very common condition appears mostly as the common cold and flu. Wind combines with heat to produce symptoms of fever, sore throat, thirst, headache, sweating, rapid pulse, and sometimes a red tip of the tongue. The treatment principle is to repel the wind and clear the heat with acupuncture and herbal formulas.

Excess Heat in the Organs: Symptoms of this yang excess condition are, typically, irritability, thirst, dry throat, concentrated (dark or burning) urine, constipation, red tongue with a yellow coat, and a full, rapid pulse (see "Diagnosis in Traditional Chinese Medicine," pages 108–126). Other symptoms depend on the organ affected. For example, heart fire produces severe emotional disturbances; stomach fire can cause mouth ulcers; liver fire might stir up extreme anger; lung fire might bring about an accumulation of yellow mucus in the lungs. In all cases, the treatment is to clear the excess heat with herbs and with manipulation of acupuncture points that have an affinity for the organ affected.

Deficiency Heat: This syndrome is caused by a deficiency in the yin, cooling aspect of an organ; the resulting imbalance causes heat to flare up. The general symptoms of deficiency heat are red cheeks, night sweats, irritability, chronic inflammation, red tongue with no coat, and a thin, rapid pulse. Other symptoms depend on the organ affected. When the kidneys have deficiency heat, chronic urinary tract infections can occur; deficiency heat in the lungs—which can arise from cigarette smoking—can lead to a chronic dry cough; and the heat from heart yin deficiency can cause insomnia.

DAMPNESS

In nature, dampness soaks the ground and everything that comes in contact with it, and stagnation results. Once something becomes damp, it can take a long time for it to dry out again, especially in wet weather. The yin pathogenic influence of dampness has similar qualities: It is persistent and heavy, and it can be difficult to resolve. A person who spends a lot of time in the rain, lives in a damp environment, or sleeps on the ground may be susceptible to external dampness. Similarly, a person who eats large amounts of ice cream, cold foods and drinks, greasy foods, and sweets is prone to imbalances of internal dampness.

Dampness has both tangible and intangible aspects. Tangible dampness includes phlegm, edema (fluid retention), and discharges. Intangible dampness includes a person's subjective feelings of heaviness and dizziness. A "slippery" pulse and a greasy tongue coating usually accompany both types of dampness. In general, symptoms of dampness in the body include water retention, swelling, feelings of heaviness, coughing or vomiting phlegm, and skin rashes that ooze or are crusty (as in eczema). Since dampness is heavy, it has a tendency to sink downward to affect the lower parts of the body: A person may experience a feeling of sinking or heaviness, and swelling frequently affects the legs. These characteristics are the opposite of wind, which has a tendency to affect the upper part of the body. When dampness combines with heat, the condition of damp heat develops, which can cause such symptoms as dark burning urine, sticky foul-smelling stools, yellow vaginal discharges, and jaundice.

Syndromes of Dampness

Wind Damp: This form of the common cold is characterized by chills, headache, afternoon fever, nausea, and diarrhea. A person may describe feeling as if a wet towel is wrapped around the head. Treatment includes moxibustion and aromatic herbs that repel wind and drain dampness.

Wind Damp Joint Pain: This condition is characterized by a dull and heavy pain and numbness that can persist in certain joints. Rheumatic pain that gets worse in damp weather is a good example of this type of imbalance. The condition tends to be chronic and resistant to treatment. Treatment with acupuncture and moxibustion can relieve the stiffness and pain. Herbs that clear wind damp, such as mulberry branches (sang zhi) and cinnamon twigs (gui zhi), are used to decrease swelling and improve circulation, following the Chinese principle of using "branches (tree limbs) to treat branches (body limbs)."

Damp and Toxins on the Skin: This condition includes any skin inflammation that also has a weepy, damp nature, such as eczema, skin ulcers, and allergic reactions that produce a discharge (skin eruptions that ooze or that are crusty). Herbs are used both internally and in the form of topical poultices.

Internal Dampness: Typically due to an imbalance in the spleen, symptoms of internal dampness include bloating, diarrhea, lack of appetite, undigested food in the stools, fatigue, and possible edema in the abdominal area. When a person coughs up mucus right after eating ice cream, it shows that a cold spleen produces dampness. Since excessive dampness in the spleen is stored in the lungs, a damp spleen can often lead to frequent colds and allergies. Treatment of internal dampness focuses on eliminating the dampness with diuretic herbs and activating the spleen with tonifying herbs.

DRYNESS

Dryness, one of the yang pernicious influences, is associated with autumn because a lack of humidity is common to that season in most parts of the world.

Dryness is a yang pernicious influence. It is associated with the autumn season due to the lack of humidity in most areas at that time of year. Its influence on the body is drying and astringent. It can easily deplete the body fluids, causing constipation, dry cough, concentrated urine, dryness in the throat and nose, thirst, and dry skin. Dryness typically enters the body through the nose and mouth, quickly affecting the lungs.

Chinese Healing Secrets

Syndromes of Dryness

External Warm Dryness: This syndrome is viewed traditionally as the leftover heat from summer teaming up with the dryness of autumn to attack the body. Symptoms include fever, headache, thirst, dry mouth, dry nose, dry eyes, dry cough with scanty mucus, red tongue, and a rapid pulse. Treatment involves the use of moistening herbs combined with herbs that repel wind. Pears are considered healing foods in conditions of dryness; they are very moistening and are readily available in the autumn season.

External Cool Dryness: Traditionally considered an illness of late autumn, this pattern has symptoms of chills, mild fever, lack of sweating, dry cough, nasal congestion, dry and itchy throat, and a wiry and floating pulse. Treatment is very similar to that for wind cold, with the addition of some moistening herbs.

Internal Dryness: In this chronic condition, the body fluids have been depleted over time. It can be both a result or cause of yin or blood deficiency, and it is more commonly seen in the elderly. In its more acute form, internal dryness can result from the depletion of body fluids due to sweating, vomiting, diarrhea, or bleeding. Prolonged internal or external heat usually has a detrimental long-term effect on body fluids, depleting them. Typical symptoms of internal dryness are dry, itchy skin, thirst, constipation, and a chronic shortage of body fluids. Treatment depends on the particular organ and vital substance affected by the imbalance. Yin or blood tonics are typically employed along with herbs that assist the body in retaining fluids.

Chinese Healing Secrets

An Organ in Disharmony

Each organ has a preferred internal environment, which supports its optimum functional abilities. The spleen is especially vulnerable to the influence of cold and dampness, for example, both in the external climate and in the diet. Since the spleen is the most important organ involved in digestion, this preference can be seen when a person eats too much cold, raw food. For example, ice cream is cold and it promotes dampness since it is both sweet and a dairy product. A person who eats too much ice cream, especially in cold weather, often has poor digestion and loose stools. When the spleen is cold and damp, it also causes the body to produce excessive mucus, which then overwhelms the lungs, leading to frequent colds, asthma, and allergies. (If you have ever coughed up mucus after eating ice cream, you have experienced the way cold produces dampness.)

On the other hand, hot, cooked foods nourish the spleen, especially when combined with warming, drying herbs such as ginger or black pepper. Eating foods such as this, especially in cold weather, leads to strong digestion, and the body produces less mucus, making the person less susceptible to colds and other respiratory ailments. If an organ's optimum functional environment is maintained, the organ will perform efficiently, contributing to the health of the entire body.

SUMMER HEAT

Summer heat is a yang pernicious influence that typically occurs in the heat and humidity of summer. It is "uprising and spread out," meaning it affects the head, causing thirst, red face, and headache, and it causes a person to lie down with the limbs spread out. The excessive sweating also leads to dark, concentrated urine, and depletion of the body's yin can occur. The extreme heat also affects the heart, leading to restlessness or even coma in severe cases such as heatstroke. When summer heat combines with dampness due to humidity and overconsumption of sugary drinks, such as soft drinks, the spleen is also affected. This leads to a loss of appetite, nausea, vomiting, diarrhea, and fatigue.

Treatment of summer heat is complex, depending on the organs and additional pathogenic factors involved. Usually, herbs are used that clear excess heat from within the body along with herbs that moisten the interior. Two common foods that are very effective in the treatment of this pattern are watermelon (xi gua) and mung beans (lu dou). There is also a point behind the knees (Weizhong, Bladder 40) associated with clearing heat; holding ice behind the knees helps the body cool down quickly. When digestive disturbances occur due to a combination of dampness and summer heat, cooling herbs are combined with herbs that clear turbid dampness, such as patchouli (huo xiang).

THE SEVEN EMOTIONS

Although the mind/body connection has been acknowledged only relatively recently in Western medicine, the interaction of emotions with the physical body is an essential aspect of traditional Chinese medicine. The seven basic emotions related to organ function are anger, joy, worry, pensiveness, sadness, fear, and shock (fright). Each organ has a corresponding emotion; imbalance of this emotion can affect the organ's function. For example, prolonged anger can lead to an imbalance in the liver. At the same time, liver imbalances can produce symptoms of anger, often leading to a self-perpetuating cycle.

In discussing the emotional aspect of the disease process, it is important to remember that it is normal to experience the full range of emotions. It is only when a particular emotion is experienced over a prolonged period or with particular intensity that it becomes a source of imbalance. It is obviously important for a person with severe emotional problems to get professional help from a trained psychotherapist. But even in these cases, the therapy is more effective when the corresponding organ imbalance is rectified.

Acupuncture is especially effective in treating disorders of the emotions. Even when it is not completely effective in treating a physical ailment, it almost always brings about a state of emotional peacefulness.

Anger

Anger is associated with the liver. By its nature, anger causes qi to rise, leading to a red face and red eyes, headaches, and dizziness. This matches the pattern of liver fire rising. Anger can also cause liver qi to "attack the spleen," producing lack of appetite, indigestion, and diarrhea (often experienced by those people who argue at the dinner table or eat while driving). In a more long-term view, suppressed anger or frustration often causes liver qi to become stagnant; this might result in depression or menstrual disorders. It is interesting to note that people who take herbs to release stagnant liver qi often experience bouts of anger as the stagnation is relieved. The anger passes as the condition clears. Similarly, anger and irritability are often the determining factor in diagnosing liver qi stagnation. Many people are relieved to know their rage has a physiologic basis. It is essential to avoid drinking coffee when treating anger-related liver disorders, as coffee heats the liver and greatly intensifies the condition.

JOY

The emotion of joy is connected with the heart. A disorder related to joy may sound perplexing, since most people want as much joy in their life as possible. The disorders from this emotion are not caused by happiness; rather, the imbalance comes from too much excitement or stimulation, or sudden good news that comes as a shock to the system. When evaluating stress levels, psychologists look at all sources of stress, both positive and negative. Clearly the death of a spouse or a job loss is a significant source of stress. However, a marriage or job promotion, while a happy occasion, is also a source of stress. A person who is constantly on the go, partying, and living a life of excess can eventually

Although it is considered a positive stressor, joy can shock the system and lead to heart imbalances.

develop heart imbalances with palpitations, anxiety, and insomnia. A person with heart imbalances may also exhibit emotional symptoms, since the heart is the seat of the spirit (shen). A person with extreme disturbances of heart shen might be seen chattering happily to himself with outbursts of laughter. Such behavior results from the heart organ's inability to provide a stable resting place for the spirit. This type of imbalance is treated with acupuncture along the heart meridian. Herbal treatments consist of formulas that nourish heart blood or yin. If heart fire disturbs the spirit, herbs that clear heat from the heart are used.

WORRY

A very common emotion in our stress-filled society, worry can deplete the energy of the spleen. This can cause digestive disturbances and eventually lead to chronic fatigue: A weakened spleen cannot efficiently turn food into qi, and the lungs are unable to extract qi from air efficiently. A person who worries too much "carries the weight of the world on her shoulders," a good description of how a person feels when her weak spleen qi leads to dampness. Treatment would include moxa and herbs that strengthen the spleen, allowing a person the energy to deal with life's problems instead of dwelling on them.

PENSIVENESS

Too much thinking or obsessing about a topic can also deplete the spleen, causing a stagnation of its qi. A person with this condition may exhibit such symptoms as poor appetite, forgetting to eat, and bloating after eating. In time, the person may develop a pale complexion from a deficiency of spleen qi. This can eventually affect the heart, causing the person to dream about the same subjects at night. Students are often affected by this imbalance; the standard treatment is use of herbs that tonify heart blood and spleen qi.

SADNESS

Sadness or grief affects the lungs, producing fatigue, shortness of breath, crying, or depression. Treatment for this condition involves acupuncture to points along the lung and kidney meridians. Often, herbal formulas are used that tonify the qi or yin of the lungs.

FEAR

The emotion of fear is related to the kidneys. This relationship can readily be seen when extreme fear causes a person to urinate uncontrollably. In children, this can also manifest as bed-wetting, which psychologists

Chinese Healing Secrets

have linked to insecurity and anxiety. Long-term anxiety due to worrying about the future can deplete the kidneys of yin, yang, and qi, eventually leading to chronic weakness. Treatment involves tonifying the kidneys with yin or yang tonics, depending on the particular symptoms.

SHOCK

A sudden shock can trigger the "fight or flight" reaction, causing imbalance.

Shock is especially debilitating to the kidneys and heart. The "fight or flight" reaction causes an excessive release of adrenaline from the adrenal glands that sit on top of the kidneys. This causes the heart to respond with palpitations, anxiety, and insomnia. Chronic stress from shock can be very debilitating to the entire system, causing a wide range of problems. Severe shock can have a long-term effect on the heart shen, as is evident in victims of post-traumatic stress syndrome. Treatment involves psychotherapy, herbs that calm the spirit and nourish the heart and kidneys, and regular acupuncture treatments.

OTHER CAUSES OF DISEASE

There are other causes of disease that don't fit within the categories of the six pernicious influences or the seven emotions.

PREDISPOSITION TO DISEASE

We inherit our prenatal qi and essence from our parents. This genetic inheritance is outside our control, and it can be the determining factor

Chinese Healing Secrets

in a number of ailments. For example, if a man's grandfather and father both died of heart disease in their 40s, he will be much more likely to develop heart disease than a person with a similar lifestyle whose ancestors lived into their 90s. It is necessary for a person with a weak inherited constitution to pursue a very healthy lifestyle to avoid disease.

POOR DIETARY HABITS

Poor dietary habits are a major cause of disease. Since food is the medicine we take most often, many illnesses can be quite difficult to treat unless changes occur in a person's diet. Some of the eating and drinking habits that can lead to disease:

Irregular Times and Amounts: It is important to consider the time it takes food to pass through the stomach. Simple fruits and vegetables can leave the stomach after about 20 minutes, while more concentrated proteins, starches, and fats may take 4 to 5 hours. If the stomach contains partially digested food when the person eats another meal, the digestive process can be seriously impaired. This would be similar to getting a small fire started with kindling and then dumping a load of logs on the fire. Even though logs are good fuel, the fledgling fire was not ready for so much fuel. Conversely, if a person waits too long between meals, secretion of digestive juices stops. This would be akin to letting the kindling go out before putting logs on the fire. We need to eat when the stomach signals true hunger.

Consumption of liquids is also an important cause of imbalance. If a person drinks a large glass of cold water after a meal, the digestive juices become diluted. (The stomach secretes just enough enzymes to digest a particular meal.) Also, the stomach needs a certain amount of heat for the chemical reactions of the digestive process to take place; cold liquids slow the reaction. It is best for the contents of the stomach to be a soup-like consistency, since too much dryness can also disturb digestion. Achieving this consistency can be accomplished by sipping liquids, preferably warm, along with a meal. In China and other Asian countries, it is common to serve soup with almost every meal. If a person desires cool water, the water should be consumed at least half an hour before a meal or three hours after a meal, when the stomach is empty.

Consuming the Wrong Types of Food: Foods have different energetic qualities; something appropriate for one type of person or climate might be unhealthy for another body type or weather pattern. For example, cold and raw foods are very healthy in hot weather or for a person who has too much internal heat. Conversely, these foods can deplete the spleen qi and yang and cause dampness in cold weather or in persons who have too much internal cold. In coastal California, for example, residents experience all four seasons in a twenty-four hour day. It might be foggy and cold in the morning, making a breakfast of hot grains or soup an appropriate choice. By midday, it can be sunny and hot, a good time to consume fruits and salads. Similarly, spicy food is appropriate for cold weather or

Cold and raw foods are very healthy in hot weather but can deplete spleen qi and yang in cold weather.

persons who are yang deficient, but it can cause imbalance in hot weather, especially in persons who have internal heat. This goes to show that no food is always healthy; it is a matter of choosing foods that match the internal and external climates. Certain foods, such as sweets or alcohol, are meant to be used infrequently and in small quantities; overconsumption can cause a wide range of problems.

Overeating or Undereating: Malnutrition due to undereating can lead to a chronic deficiency of qi and blood. While more common in developing countries, this condition is also seen in developed countries in conditions of poverty and in persons who suffer from emotional imbalances and substance abuse. Treatment includes herbs that tonify qi and blood, along with an improvement in nutritional intake. In the West, overconsumption is a far more common problem, leading to a high incidence of heart disease, high blood pressure, stroke, diabetes, and cancer. In traditional Chinese medicine, acupuncture is used to reduce cravings; dietary and lifestyle counseling are also important.

Food Cravings and Addictions: The human body is designed to process a wide variety of foods to meet our needs. Fad diets or addictions to a narrow range of foods can be debilitating. Some essential nutrients are likely to be missing from a narrow diet. By eating a wide assortment of different-colored vegetables, whole grains, and proteins, we can receive the nutrition we need to function at a high level of wellness.

Contaminated Food: Although more common in developing or tropical countries, parasites are a problem all over the world. They can wreak havoc on the digestive organs, damaging the qi of the spleen and stomach. Herbs that kill parasites are quite strong, so it is important to have an accurate diagnosis through a stool test before beginning treatment.

Other sources of contamination are toxins produced by bacterial contamination in the course of processing food. Meats are especially susceptible to this sort of pathogen; you should always cook meat thoroughly to kill virulent microorganisms. Water-borne pathogens are another source of disease, and water of questionable quality should always be boiled. Treatment of pathogenic microorganisms depends on the type of pathogen involved. In general, gastrointestinal distress caused by microorganisms can be treated with herbal medicines. Although herb formulas can be remarkably effective, they should be considered a first-aid measure until a person can see their health care practitioner.

Lack of Exercise

Too little exercise can lead to stagnation of qi and blood and, subsequently, a variety of degenerative diseases, including obesity, cancer, and heart disease. Moderate exercise strengthens the heart and lungs and stimulates the flow of blood and lymph, the body's filtration system, which filters out toxins. In fact, exercise is the only way to pump lymph through the body, since lymph isn't powered by the heart. Some of the traditional Chinese ideas about lack of exercise are expressed in the ancient texts:

"Sleeping or lying down too much hurts the qi." When a person oversleeps, he typically feels tired all day.

"Too much sitting hurts the muscles." This refers to the fact that lack of exercise causes the muscles to atrophy.

"A running stream doesn't go bad." Stagnant water easily becomes spoiled, and stagnant qi and blood can lead to many different illnesses.

On the other hand, too much activity can hurt the body. This is especially true if a person is fighting a cold or is already depleted and in need of rest. In these cases, almost any exercise can drain the qi. Some of the traditional ideas about excessive activity:

"Using the eyes too much hurts the blood." Since the eyes are intimately connected with the liver, excessive use of the eyes can drain that

Chinese Healing Secrets

organ. The liver stores the blood, so stressing it in this way depletes the blood supply.

"Too much standing hurts the bones." People who must stand all day at work, especially on a concrete floor, can vouch for the truth of this statement. Some of the conditions that can be caused by standing too much are sore feet, painful joints, and varicose veins.

Standing all day, especially on hard surfaces, tends to cause sore feet, painful joints, and varicose veins.

"Too much walking hurts the tendons." Tendinitis is a very common condition, especially among runners. Computer work and repetitive stress injuries are also frequent causes of tendon injury.

"Too much work for the heart injures the spirit (shen)." Since the heart is the seat of the mind, too much mental work affects the spirit. It is important to get sufficient physical exercise to avoid this imbalance.

"Too much work for the liver hurts the blood." The liver blood can also be depleted by too much work, as can be seen in marathon runners who no longer have menstrual periods. When they ease up on their workouts, their menstrual periods usually return.

"Too much work for the kidneys hurts the essence (jing)." Each individual has a different capacity for sexual activity, depending on their age and their constitution. Overindulgence in sexual activity, however, can lead to a depletion of the kidneys, causing fatigue and chronic pain in the low back.

ACCIDENTS AND INJURIES

These causes of disease are self-explanatory. However, a person with strong qi and blood will recover from injuries much faster than a person who is deficient in these vital substances. Traditional Chinese medicine is especially effective in treating injuries of all types.

SIDE EFFECTS OF MEDICAL TREATMENTS

This is especially common with Western medicine, where the list of possible side effects for a drug might fill two pages of text. A recent study found that in some hospitals, as many as 30 percent of patients at any given time are receiving treatment for the side effects of the drugs they're taking. Herbal medicine can be very helpful in reducing many of these side effects; cancer patients in Chinese hospitals, for example, are routinely prescribed herbs to help counteract the side effects of chemotherapy.

Although herbal medicine is exceptionally safe, side effects can occur, although they are rarely serious. For example, many herbs are hard to digest and can cause loose stools. An herbalist takes this into account when preparing a formula for a patient, adding specific herbs to counteract these side effects.

If herbs are improperly prescribed, on the other hand, the side effects can be more severe. For example, a person who suffers from high blood pressure should never be given the herb *Ephedra* (ma huang), since it can cause a rise in blood pressure. For this reason, traditional Chinese medical texts also list formulas that are used to counteract the effects of improper treatments.

CHAPTER 6:
Disorders of the
Internal Organs

Once a practitioner establishes a general diagnosis, taking into account the eight parameters, the vital substances, and the pernicious influences, the next step is to determine which organ systems are affected. This logical procedure leads to a final diagnosis that is specific enough to enable the physician to prepare a focused treatment plan. For example, a patient may have chronic night sweats, irritability, and thirst—general signs of yin deficiency—but the practitioner still does not know which organ system to nourish at this point. Keeping in mind the normal functions of the organs, the practitioner might find further symptoms of palpitations, insomnia, and poor memory, concluding that the yin deficiency affects mostly the heart. The treatment plan would then include an herbal formula to nourish heart yin.

It is rare when all of the classic symptoms of a typical syndrome are present. In fact, it is more common for just a few symptoms to occur, and these often arise from two or three simultaneous disease patterns. For example, a person might have chronic spleen qi deficiency with symptoms of only poor appetite and loose stools. The same person could also have liver qi stagnation with the only symptom being pre-menstrual syndrome once a month. If this person catches a cold on top of these underlying disorders, her symptoms would involve three separate patterns of disharmony. Early-stage and mild versions of syndromes may have very subtle symptom patterns; these require the diagnostic skills of an experienced practitioner.

It is important to remember that the functions of organs in traditional Chinese medicine may overlap those of their Western counterparts, but they also have totally unrelated functions. For this reason, it is dangerous to attempt to find a standard correspondence between the two. For example, a chest cold might be diagnosed as a lung condition under both systems, but asthma might be a kidney condition in traditional Chinese medical diagnostics. Both medical systems stand on their own strengths, but an attempt to artificially link the two can often make them less effective. Attempting to treat the flu simply with Chinese herbs that have antiviral qualities is less effective than getting an accurate diagnosis—wind heat, for example—and using a traditional formula for that wind heat.

The following section briefly describes the various conditions of imbalance that make up the foundation for an effective traditional treatment plan. Please keep in mind that many of these descriptions are for severe versions of the syndromes. The description of each pattern lists the full range of severity, from a mild set of symptoms to life-threatening disease. If intervention takes place at the early stages, it is possible to restore balance before the symptoms become more severe.

LUNG SYNDROMES

The lungs are in direct contact with the external environment; therefore, they are the organ most subject to attacks by external pernicious influences. They are also prone to disorders of yin deficiency and dryness, due to their need for a somewhat moist environment to function. (Each organ has its "favorite" climate, and a moist environment helps the lungs function.) Since the lungs govern qi, they affect the energy of the entire body if they become qi deficient.

Chinese Healing Secrets

Lung Qi Deficiency: This syndrome is characterized by shortness of breath, weak voice, spontaneous sweating, chronic weak cough, fatigue, bright pale face, frequent colds, a weak pulse, and a pale tongue. Some corresponding Western conditions might be asthma, emphysema, chronic bronchitis, allergies, depressed immune function, AIDS, and cancer. The treatment principle is to tonify lung qi with herbs such as ginseng (ren shen) and *Astragalus* (huang qi).

Lung Yin Deficiency: A chronic deficiency pattern, lung yin deficiency produces such symptoms as night sweats, low-grade fever, dry cough, small amounts of sticky phlegm or no phlegm, dry mouth, thirst, red cheeks, vocal distortions (weak voice, hoarseness, pitch changes), heat in the "five palms" (palms, soles, and sternum), red tongue with little or no coat, and a small rapid pulse. Western diagnoses are smoker's cough, tuberculosis, chronic sore throat, or chronic bronchitis. Treatment is to tonify lung yin and clear deficiency heat with herbs such as *Rehmannia* (sheng di huang) or *Ophiopogon* (mai men dong).

Wind Cold: This acute excess syndrome produces chills, possibly a mild fever, nasal congestion, headaches, upper body aches, a cough with clear or white phlegm that is easy to expectorate, and a tight, floating pulse. The common cold, acute bronchitis, and the early stages of pneumonia are considered to be wind cold conditions in traditional Chinese medicine. The treatment principle is to "release the exterior" with warm, diaphoretic herbs such as *Ephedra* (ma huang).

The common cold is considered to be a wind cold condition. Warm, diaphoretic herbs are used to treat it.

Wind Heat: This acute pattern differs somewhat from wind cold due to the influence of heat. Symptoms include a fever worse than the chills, a loud cough with yellow phlegm, sore throat, and a rapid, floating pulse. Treatment involves cooling herbs that release the exterior, such as honeysuckle (jin yin hua) or field mint (bo he).

Damp Phlegm Blocking the Lung: Copious amounts of clear or white phlegm is the main symptom of this excess syndrome. Other symptoms are shortness of breath, fullness in the chest, a thick, greasy tongue coating, slippery pulse, and a worsening of the symptoms when lying down. Corresponding Western conditions are chronic bronchitis with an acute episode, asthma, and bronchiectasis. Treatment involves herbs that clear phlegm from the lungs such as *Pinellia* (ban xia).

Hot Phlegm Stagnation: A serious internal excess pattern, hot phlegm stagnation produces such symptoms as difficulty breathing, thirst, a loud, frequent cough with green-yellow or bloody phlegm, a fishy smell on the breath, constipation, dark urine, chest pain, high fever, red tongue with a thick yellow coat, and a slippery, rapid pulse. Western diagnoses could be lung abscess, acute bronchitis, or pneumonia. Cooling antibiotic herbs, such as *Houttuynia* (yu xing cao) and *Scutellaria* (huang qin), are used.

Dryness Attacking the Lung: Symptoms of this syndrome include a dry cough, dry and cracked tongue coat, loss of voice, dry nose, sore, dry throat, and a floating, rapid pulse. Although it shares some aspects of yin deficiency, dryness attacking the lung is acute and external, while yin deficiency is chronic and internal. Another distinguishing factor is the lack of deficiency heat signs such as night sweats and "five palm heat." Some corresponding Western conditions are the common cold, acute bronchitis, later-stage pneumonia, allergy, and dehydration due to an overly dry environment. Herbs that moisten the lungs and release the exterior, such as *Phragmites* (lu gen) and kudzu (ge gen), are used.

SPLEEN SYNDROMES

The main functions of the spleen are to transform food and fluids, nourish the muscles, and control the blood, keeping it within the blood vessels. For this reason, most patterns of disharmony of the spleen involve poor appetite and digestion, fatigue, and bleeding disorders. The spleen prefers a dry environment, so it is prone to conditions of dampness from climate and dietary factors. It is especially sensitive to cold, damp weather and cold or raw foods, both of which are fertile ground for the pathogenic factor of dampness. When the spleen functions properly, the body is strong and well nourished. Blood, fluids, and the organs are also in their proper places; thus there is no deficient-type bleeding (blood), edema (fluids), or prolapse (organs).

Spleen Qi Deficiency: When the qi of the spleen is deficient, the spleen is unable to perform its functions of digestion. In addition to the typical qi deficiency signs of fatigue and pale face and tongue, additional symptoms specific to the spleen include poor appetite, weight loss, fullness and sleepiness after eating, and loose stools. (Other conditions are associated with spleen qi deficiency, such as sagging organs and bleeding, but these are discussed as separate syndromes.) Some corresponding Western conditions are ulcers, gastritis, chronic fatigue, AIDS, chronic indigestion, and hepatitis. Treatment consists of tonifying spleen qi with herbs such as ginseng (ren shen). The classic formula to tonify spleen qi is Four Gentlemen decoction (Si Jun Zi Tang).

Spleen Yang Deficiency: This more severe version of spleen qi deficiency has the above-mentioned symptoms as well as cold signs such as cold hands and feet, edema, a desire for warm food and drinks, abdominal discomfort after eating cold food, and diarrhea with undigested food in the stools. Western diseases that fit this syndrome are chronic gastroenteritis, infection with *Candida*, food allergies, and chronic hepatitis. The treatment principle is to tonify spleen qi and yang and warm the interior with herbs such as ginseng (ren shen), *Astragalus* (huang qi), ginger (gan jiang), and black pepper (hu jiao).

Abdominal discomfort that occurs after eating cold foods, such as ice cream, is a sign of spleen yang deficiency.

Spleen Qi Collapse or Spleen Qi Sinking: Since spleen qi supports the organs with its uplifting energy, this aspect of deficient qi is associated with a prolapse (sagging) and a sensation of bearing down in the internal organs. Some organs affected are the stomach, transverse colon, uterus, and rectum. Hemorrhoids are also a condition of spleen qi collapse. In some cases, miscarriages can occur from lack of qi to "hold things up," or retain the fetus with "upward" force. Treatment is to "raise the middle qi" with classic formulas such as Bu Zhong Yi Qi Tang ("Decoction to Tonify the Middle Burner and Raise the Vital Energy"). This formula contains herbs such as ginseng (ren shen) and *Astragalus* (huang qi) to build the spleen qi, along with herbs that have an uplifting energy such as *Bupleurum* (chai hu) and *Cimicifuga* (sheng ma).

Spleen Not Controlling the Blood: Another function of spleen qi is to keep the blood flowing within the vessels. When this function is disturbed, standard symptoms of spleen qi deficiency occur along with bleeding under the skin (easy bruising), excessive menstrual bleeding, nosebleeds, and blood in the urine or stools. Since this bleeding is due to deficiency, the color of the blood is often lighter than might occur in excess bleeding disorders such as heat in the blood. Some of the Western disease patterns that could fall into this pattern are any chronic bleeding diseases, hemophilia, bleeding hemorrhoids, bruising from vitamin deficiency, and periodontal disease. The treatment is to tonify spleen qi and tonify blood. The classic formula for this purpose, Eight Treasure Decoction (Ba Zhen Tang), combines the standard formulas for qi and blood tonification.

Cold and Damp Surrounding the Spleen: This excess pattern arises when the dampness pernicious influence overwhelms the spleen. Symptoms include abdominal fullness and bloating, nausea, vomiting, watery stool, lack of thirst, sticky sensation and sweet taste in the mouth, dizziness, heavy feelings in the body, and a thick, greasy coat on the tongue. Some corresponding Western conditions are stomach "flu," chronic gastritis, chronic colitis, ulcers, and hepatitis. The treatment involves the use of fragrant herbs that "penetrate the dampness and wake up the spleen," such as patchouli (huo xiang).

Damp Heat in the Spleen: In this excess disharmony condition, the dampness symptoms combine with those of heat. They are: jaundice, yellow eyes, bitter taste in the mouth, nausea, vomiting, dislike of greasy food, burning urine and diarrhea, abdominal pain, bloating, and mouth sores. Some Western diagnoses are hepatitis, gallbladder disease, and acute gastroenteritis. The treatment principle is to clear damp heat with herbs such as *Coptis* (huang lian) and *Artemisia* (yin chen hao).

HEART SYNDROMES

The heart governs the blood and vessels and is the seat of the mind and spirit. Disorders of the heart tend to involve emotional and mental disturbances as well as some circulatory conditions such as cold hands and feet. Generally, external pernicious influences don't affect the heart directly; instead, they typically attack the pericardium, the sac around the heart known in Chinese medicine as the "heart protector." In almost all disharmonies of the heart, palpitations are a key symptom. This pounding of the heart occurs in both excess and deficiency patterns.

Heart Qi Deficiency: Palpitations are the key symptom in this deficiency pattern. Other symptoms are spontaneous sweating (sweating without exertion or overheating), physical and mental fatigue, depression, pale face, and a weak pulse, especially in the heart area on the left wrist. This pattern can correspond to chronic fatigue, neurasthenia (chronic mental and physical weakness), or heart disease involving the muscle, valves, or vessels. The treatment principle for this deficiency is to tonify heart qi with standard qi tonics such as ginseng (ren shen), along with herbs that act specifically on the heart, such as *Schizandra* (wu wei zi) and *Biota* (bai zi ren).

Heart Yang Deficiency: This syndrome has all the symptoms of heart qi deficiency with the addition of cold symptoms: feeling cold in the limbs or entire body; purple face, tongue, and lips due to cold stagnating the circulation; and a slow, choppy, and intermittent pulse. A deeper, more serious condition than qi deficiency, heart yang deficiency typically corresponds to a Western diagnosis of true heart disease. The treatment is to tonify heart yang with moxibustion and herbs such as ginseng (ren shen) and aconite (fu zi). **Note:** Aconite is a highly toxic herb, and it should only be used in a formula prepared and supervised by a qualified practitioner of traditional Chinese medicine.

Heart Yang Collapse: A more severe version of heart yang deficiency, heart yang collapse produces all the symptoms of qi and yang deficiency plus copious cold sweats, extreme cold in the limbs, very weak breathing, a minute pulse, and abnormal shen that precedes a comatose state. Corresponding Western diagnoses are shock or heart attack, so this syndrome requires hospitalization. In China, the person receives herbal treatment while hospitalized. Typical treatment is an intravenous drip of *Salvia* (dan shen) and oral doses of ginseng (ren shen) and aconite (fu zi).

When heart blood is deficient, there is no calm foundation for the spirit, and the result is insomnia.

Heart Blood Deficiency: This pattern of deficiency involving the blood produces symptoms of palpitations, fearfulness and a propensity to be easily startled, insomnia, excessive dreams while asleep, mental restlessness, forgetfulness, dizziness, pale face and tongue, and a thin, small pulse. The insomnia is due to an insufficient amount of blood to provide a calm foundation for the spirit. Possibly corresponding to anemia or emotional imbalances, this deficiency syndrome is treated by tonifying heart blood with herbs such as *Angelica sinensis* (dang gui) and longan fruit (long yan rou).

Heart Yin Deficiency: This syndrome of deficiency heat produces red cheeks, night sweats, "five palm heat," dry mouth, thirst for small amounts of water, mental restlessness, insomnia, palpitations, low-grade fever, forgetfulness, excessive dreaming, red tongue with little or no coat, and a small, rapid pulse. A person with this deficiency has difficulty remaining asleep—the heat condition wakes them. Because the heart is the seat of the spirit, an insufficiency of calming, nurturing yin or blood in the heart results in agitation. Hypertension and hyperthyroidism can match this pattern, which is treated with herbs that clear heat and tonify heart yin such as Emperor's Teapills (Tian Wang Bu Xin Dan).

Heart Fire Uprising: This excess heat pattern produces symptoms that include a red face, dry mouth with a desire for lots of water, a red tip and prickles on the tongue with possible ulcers and pain, bitter taste in the mouth, burning urine, mental restlessness, insomnia, and a full, rapid pulse. Excess heat signs are stronger than those of heat due to yin deficiency. Some corresponding Western conditions are urinary tract infection, high blood pressure, or tongue infection. The treatment aims to clear heat and calm the spirit with acupuncture and herbs such as lotus seed sprouts (lian zi xin) and *Coptis* (huang lian).

Heart Blood Stagnation: This serious heart condition has symptoms of a sharp, stabbing pain in the heart area, pain that can radiate up the arm, purple face and tongue, fatigue, palpitations, and a choppy, wiry, or intermittent pulse. It sometimes occurs with heart yang or qi deficiency and includes the symptoms common to these patterns. Corresponding Western diseases are angina pectoris, coronary arteriosclerosis, or pericarditis—all requiring intensive medical intervention. Treatment involves regulating the qi and vitalizing the blood with circulatory stimulants such as *Salvia* (dan shen) and *Panax pseudoginseng* (san qi).

Hot Phlegm Confusing the Heart: This excess condition is characterized by excess heat causing a red face and eyes, irrational and possibly violent behavior, nonstop loud talking, anger, a red tongue with a greasy yellow coat, and a rapid, slippery pulse. It corresponds to the Western diagnoses of mental illness, mania, or encephalitis. The treatment for hot phlegm confusing the heart is to calm the spirit and clear heat and phlegm with acupuncture and herbs such as *Coptis* (huang lian) and *Borneol* (bing pian).

Phlegm Misting the Heart Opening: In this condition, which is related to the above syndrome but with less heat, symptoms include a pale tongue with a white coating, mental confusion, difficulty speaking (muttering to oneself, drooling), the sound of phlegm in the throat, and possible loss of consciousness. Some corresponding Western diseases are stroke, epilepsy, mental retardation, or mental illness. The treatment principle is to clear the phlegm and revive the consciousness with scalp acupuncture and herbs that resolve phlegm and wake up the spirit, such as *Calamus* (shi chang pu).

PERICARDIUM SYNDROMES

The pericardium is considered the sixth yin organ, but its functions are typically linked with the heart. The shield between the heart and the exterior, the pericardium protects the heart from the invasion of external pathogenic factors. Its main syndrome is known as "heat crushing the pericardium," which is characterized by a high fever, mental confusion, convulsions, and, possibly, coma. This pattern can appear in acute febrile diseases with a high fever, such as encephalitis or pericarditis, where the sudden high temperature affects the consciousness. Treatment includes the use of acupuncture points on the pericardium meridian, along with herbs that clear excess heat, such as tree peony root (mu dan pi).

LIVER SYNDROMES

Imbalances of the liver are seen commonly in clinical practice, since the stress and toxicity of modern life (poor diet, chemicals in our food and environment, stress, overwork, etc.) take a toll on this organ. Since

the liver plays the central role in the smooth flow of qi and emotion in the body, disharmony of the liver can affect any of the other organs. Typically, disorders of the menstrual cycle or stress-related ailments indicate a problem with the liver.

Polution in the environment takes a toll on the liver. Imbalances in the liver can, in turn, affect any of the other organs of the body.

Liver Qi Stagnation: This is one of the most common diagnoses in traditional Chinese medicine. When the qi of the liver is stuck, symptoms of frustration, irritability, depression, anxiety, fullness in the chest, menstrual disorders, and indigestion can occur. This excess condition can also arise in a person who has experienced long-term depression or frustrations, creating a vicious cycle of cause and effect. Some Western conditions that fit this pattern are premenstrual syndrome, depression, hepatitis, or chronic fatigue. Treatment with acupuncture often has an immediate effect in relieving the symptoms. A classic formula known as Xiao Yao Wan ("Free and Easy Wanderer Pills") is also very effective in rectifying this liver syndrome.

Liver Fire Uprising: This excess heat pattern mainly affects the upper body, since heat rises naturally. The entire face is red, with additional

火 Life Out of Balance

Joe is a 40-year-old executive with a high-stress lifestyle, often working overtime. He drinks coffee frequently to "keep up his energy," and his meals often consist of pastries from a vending machine. His colleagues complain he is prone to bouts of sudden anger for no good reason, so they keep their distance. He always seems to have a stiff neck, and his face and eyes are often red. His doctor is very concerned about his high blood pressure, and his wife has warned him that she will leave him if he doesn't stop yelling at her at the slightest provocation.

This is a classic case of excess liver yang or fire, caused by Joe's lifestyle and diet. The symptoms can be alleviated with acupuncture and herbal therapy. However, to achieve lasting healing, Joe's life needs a major overhaul. In addition to working less, the most important change he must make is to eliminate coffee, since it directly overheats the liver. Since caffeine withdrawal can also cause similar symptoms, green tea is a good substitute at first. Although it still has some caffeine, green tea has a cooling energy that disturbs the liver far less. And it can be decreased or eliminated later without causing discomfort. A well-balanced diet is also essential, since a deficient diet harms the liver and also leads to qi deficiency and a consequent craving for stimulants. Exercise and stress-reduction techniques will also help lower blood pressure and create an appetite for good food. Once Joe's liver cools down with lifestyle changes, acupuncture, and herbal therapy, he will be much less prone to outbursts of anger. He can then take cooling tonics such as American ginseng, which will give him extra energy without creating all the side effects of coffee.

signs and symptoms of red eyes, anger, headache, ringing in the ears (tinnitus), bitter taste in the mouth, insomnia, constipation, dark urine, red tongue with a yellow coat, and a full, rapid pulse. The condition can arise from long-term stagnation of qi due to anger, alcoholism, or chronic liver imbalances that develop into heat patterns. Some corre-

Chinese Healing Secrets

sponding Western diagnoses are hypertension, alcoholism, hyperthyroidism, acute hepatitis, gallbladder infection, ear infection, and conjunctivitis. Treatment involves clearing heat and regulating the liver with acupuncture and herbal formulas such as Long Dan Xie Gan Wan.

Liver and Gallbladder Damp Heat: When dampness accumulates in the body and combines with heat in the liver and gallbladder, this excess syndrome develops. Its symptoms are jaundice and dark urine, which are caused by a stagnation of yellow bile that backs up and is excreted through the skin and urine. Additional symptoms include a lack of appetite, an aversion to greasy food, digestive problems, bitter taste in the mouth, nausea, vomiting, burning diarrhea, a red tongue with a thick, greasy yellow coat, and a slippery, rapid pulse. In Western medicine, most of these symptoms are typical of acute hepatitis or gallbladder infections, but this pattern can also correspond to herpes, vaginal discharges, testicular pain, and eczema. The treatment principle is to clear heat and drain dampness with herbs such as rhubarb root (da huang), gentian (long dan cao), and *Artemisia* (yin chen hao).

Liver Wind Moving Internally: Since the liver is in charge of the smooth flow of qi, any abnormal body movements are typically related to liver imbalances due to wind. This internal wind is considered an excess pattern, but it can arise from a variety of causes, such as blood deficiency, excess heat, or liver yin deficiency. The cardinal symptoms involve abnormal movements such as shaking, spasms, tics, rigidity, and convulsions. Dizziness, headache, and difficulty in speaking may also occur. The tongue and pulse signs depend on which underlying pattern has caused the stirring of wind, but the pulse is usually wiry, a typical sign of liver imbalance. This pattern is seen in stroke patients and those

Chrysanthemum, or jua hua, is used in the treatment of liver wind moving internally.

with Parkinson disease and cases of seizures associated with a high fever, tetanus, and hypertension. Acupuncture can be a very effective treatment, as are herbs that clear liver wind and heat, such as *Gastrodia* (tian ma), *Uncaria* (gou teng), and *Chrysanthemum* (jua hua). If the problem is caused by depletion, the underlying deficiency must be tonified. For example, if wind is due to deficient liver yin, treatment must both tonify the liver yin and subdue the wind.

Cold Stagnation in the Liver Channel: The liver meridian encircles the genital area, so localized disorders in the reproductive organs are often traced to a blockage in that meridian. This syndrome is characterized by pain in the groin, lower abdomen, and testicles and is relieved by application of heat. This pattern typically corresponds to a hernia but may also be present in cold-type menstrual disorders and infertility. Treatment involves warming with moxa and using herbs that regulate qi and warm the liver meridian, such as *Galangal* (gao liang jiang) and lychee seed (li zhi he).

Liver Blood Deficiency: This syndrome has the typical symptoms of blood deficiency: pale face and tongue, dizziness, dry skin, and thin pulse. The condition of the eyes and nails are clues to the state of the liver, so symptoms may include pale, cracked nails, blurred vision, itchy eyes, night blindness, and visual distortions such as spots and floaters. Menstrual flow may be scanty or nonexistent, and lack of nourishment to the tendons from liver blood deficiency can lead to pain, numbness, or cramping in the legs. Possible Western diagnoses are anemia, malnutrition, hypertension, menstrual disorders, and eye problems. Treatment involves tonifying the blood with standard blood tonics such as *Angelica sinensis* (dang gui), cooked *Rehmannia* (shu di huang), and *Polygonum multiflorum* (he shou wu), along with herbs that specifically nourish the liver such as *Lycium* fruit (gou qi zi).

Liver Yin Deficiency: This syndrome exhibits the usual signs of "five palm heat": red cheeks, night sweats, red tongue with no coat, and a thin, rapid pulse. Additional symptoms specific to the liver are dizziness, irritability, and dry, irritated eyes. Treatment involves tonifying liver yin and clearing heat with formulas such as Chrysanthemum, Lycium, and Rehmannia Pills (Qi Ju Di Huang Wan).

Liver Yang Rising: If liver yin deficiency continues without treatment, the deficiency heat rises to the head. Known as liver yang rising, it produces additional symptoms of headache and anger. It is an intermediate syndrome—more severe than a simple yin deficiency but less severe than liver fire. Some Western diagnoses are anemia, chronic hepatitis, hypertension, eye problems, menopause, and menstrual disorders. Treatment involves sedating the excess liver yang with formulas such as Gastrodia and Uncaria Combination (Tian Ma Gou Teng Yin). If the yang rising symptoms are especially severe, heavy herbs that settle yang, such as oyster shell (mu li), are added.

KIDNEY SYNDROMES

Since the kidneys are the source of yin and yang for the entire body, a kidney imbalance can have an effect anywhere in the body. They are the storage site for the essence, the substance responsible for growth, fertility, and vitality, so the kidneys are only subject to syndromes of deficiency. Patterns of deficient qi, yin, or yang are often traced to a corresponding syndrome of deficiency within the kidneys; similarly, a long-term depletion in any organ eventually depletes the kidneys.

Kidney Yang Deficiency: The kidney yang is the source of metabolic fire (the heat needed for digestion and other bodily functions) for the entire body. When kidney yang is depleted, symptoms are cold hands and feet, frequent urination with clear urine or water retention and edema, night urination, pallor, pain in the lower back and knees, low sex drive, apathy, and an aversion to cold environments. This chronic condition can correspond to the Western conditions of

Cinnamon bark may be used to treat kidney yang deficieny.

nephritis, hypothyroidism, adrenal insufficiency, chronic low back pain, depression, and sexual dysfunction. Treatment involves tonifying the "life-gate fire" by applying heat from moxibustion at a point below the second lumbar vertebra. The standard herb formula is Rehmannia Eight (Ba Wei Di Huang Wan), which contains herbs that nourish the kidneys along with hot metabolic stimulants such as cinnamon bark (rou gui) and aconite (fu zi).

Kidney Yang Deficiency with Dirty Water Flooding: This syndrome exhibits all the above symptoms of yang deficiency, but in this case the lack of yang leads to a debility in fluid transformation (fluids don't move to their proper locations; instead, they collect in organs or limbs). The specific symptoms related to this metabolic failure include edema in the lower body, abdominal fullness, nausea, difficulty breathing, cough or asthma with thin mucus, and small amounts of clear urine.

This syndrome can correspond to congestive heart failure or nephritis. Treatment consists of tonifying kidney yang as above, with the addition of diuretic herbs such as *Plantago* seeds (che qian zi) and ginger root skin (sheng jiang pi).

Kidney Yin Deficiency: This condition of deficiency heat is due to a depletion of the yin. Typical yin deficiency signs of red cheeks, night sweats, "five palm heat," dry mouth, a red tongue with little or no coat, and a thin, rapid pulse occur. In addition, depletion symptoms specific to the kidneys occur, such as concentrated urine, nocturnal emissions of semen, premature ejaculation, overactive sex drive, vertigo, ringing in the ears, insomnia, and sore low back and knees. This pattern might match Western diagnoses of lumbago, hypertension, diabetes, hyperthyroidism, and psychological or emotional disorders. The standard base formula for all varieties of kidney yin deficiency is Rehmannia Teapills (Liu Wei Di Huang Wan).

Kidney Essence (Jing) Deficiency: The kidney essence is responsible for growth, development, and reproduction. Children with this deficiency may exhibit late closure of the soft spots in the skull, slow growth, late development of speech and walking, or mental retardation. Adults may experience premature aging, fragile bones, loss of teeth and hair, infertility, and poor memory. In children, the syndrome is entirely genetic; in adults the pattern arises from old age or "burning the candle at both ends." Treatment consists of tonifying kidney yin and yang; the balance of warm and cold herbs is tailored to fit the individual situation. In addition, herbs are used that specifically strengthen the essence, such as privet fruit (nu zhen zi) and *Cuscuta* (tu si zi).

SMALL INTESTINE SYNDROMES

The small intestine's functions are to separate food and fluids into essential and waste components. A yang organ, its patterns of disharmony are usually related to a dysfunction in a yin organ such as the heart or spleen.

Small Intestine Deficient and Cold: This pattern can arise in a deficiency of spleen yang. Symptoms include pain around the navel that is relieved with pressure and heat, watery diarrhea or loose stools, frequent clear urination, and a gurgling sound in the abdomen. The tongue is pale with a white coat, and the pulse is deep, empty, and slow. Some corresponding Western conditions are infections with the *Candida* organism, food allergies, enteritis, chronic dysentery, or stress-related digestive disorders. Treatment involves tonifying spleen yang with moxibustion and warm, strengthening herbs such as ginseng (ren shen) and ginger (gan jiang).

Small Intestine Excess Heat: Excess heat in the heart can be transferred to the small intestine, since the two organs are paired in a yin/yang relationship. When this occurs, the symptoms include frequent dark burning urine, thirst, a red tip on the tongue, mental restlessness, and a rapid, full pulse. Although the cause is often emotional hyperactivity, the excess heat shows up in the urine in a typical Western diagnosis of urinary tract infection. The treatment principle is to clear heat from the heart and small intestine with acupuncture and herbs such as *Lophatherum* (dan zhu ye) and lotus sprout (lian zi xin).

Small Intestine Qi Pain: Often associated with stagnant liver qi, this pattern exhibits distention and pain in the lower abdomen that feels worse when pressure is applied, distention and pain in the groin, gurgling sounds in the abdominal area, pain relief after passing gas, a pale tongue with a thin, white coat, and a deep, wiry pulse. Corresponding Western conditions might be hernia of the small intestine, colitis, food allergies, and enteritis. Since it is a disorder of stagnant qi, acupuncture and stress reduction are particularly helpful to treat it. Herbal therapy includes herbs to regulate qi, such as *Bupleurum* (chai hu), white peony root (bai shao), and *Cyperus* (xiang fu).

LARGE INTESTINE SYNDROMES

The large intestine has the same functions in traditional Chinese medicine as it does in Western physiology: receiving food from the small intestine, separating the fluids, and passing on the remainder as waste. Dysfunctions of the large intestine typically involve a disruption in one of these activities, often due to poor dietary habits.

Large Intestine Excess Heat: This excess syndrome is characterized by constipation, a bloated, painful abdomen, fever, explosive burning diarrhea with a bad smell, concentrated urine, thirst, a red tongue with a thick yellow coat, and a full, rapid pulse. It is associated with acute bacterial dysentery or any serious infection. Treatment involves clearing excess heat from the large intestine with cooling purgative herbs such as rhubarb (da huang) and *Mirabilite* (mang xiao).

Large Intestine Damp Heat: This pattern is similar to the excess heat syndrome described above, with the addition of the influence of dampness, which makes recovery slower than with simple excess heat. The dampness also creates the additional symptoms of fatigue, a sensation of not being finished when defecating, blood or pus in the stools, intermittent fever, a slippery pulse, and a greasy yellow tongue coating.

This pattern corresponds to acute amoebic dysentery or hemorrhoids and is treated with herbs that clear dampness and heat from the large intestine, such as *Coptis* (huang lian) and *Pulsatilla* (bai tou weng).

Large Intestine Closed and Knotted: This excess pattern has symptoms of abdominal bloating with pain that gets worse when pressure is applied, constipation, nausea, vomiting, deep, full pulse, and a greasy, thick white coat on the tongue. It is seen in intestinal blockages due to a hernia or scar tissue and is often seen in children. Typically, surgery is required. If the blockage is only partial, acupuncture and strong purgative herbs such as *Croton* (ba dou) can alleviate the symptoms.

Heat Stagnation in the Large Intestine: This excess pattern, which combines excess heat with qi and blood stagnation, causes sharp, fixed abdominal pain that worsens when pressure is applied, bloating, constipation or diarrhea, vomiting, fever, a deep-red tongue with a thick yellow dry coat, and a full, wiry, rapid pulse. Possible Western diagnoses are appendicitis, diverticulitis, and some dysentery. This is a serious condition, and proper medical intervention is essential. An acupuncture point on the leg known as Lanwei is specific for appendicitis. Since this condition can be caused by hardened feces blocking the appendix, stimulating this point could dislodge the blockage, explaining this point's effectiveness in treating early-stage appendicitis. Treatment includes cooling, purgative herbs such as rhubarb root (da huang) and herbs such as tree peony root (mu dan pi) to move stagnant qi and blood.

Large Intestine Fluid Deficiency: The fluid deficiency in this syndrome can arise from old age, dehydration after an illness, delivery of a baby, or chronic infections. The symptoms are chronic constipation, dry mouth,

Herbal prescriptions are generally tailored to the needs of the individual.

dry stools, small and rapid pulse, and a dry, red, and cracked tongue. The treatment principle for this syndrome is to clear heat and moisten the intestines with herbs such as *Cannabis* seeds (huo ma ren) and *Rehmannia* root (sheng di huang).

Large Intestine Deficient and Cold: Usually a result of spleen yang deficiency, this pattern has symptoms of watery diarrhea without a strong smell, abdominal pain relieved by pressure and warmth, gurgling abdominal sounds, a worsening of symptoms after eating cold food, deep weak pulse, and a pale, swollen tongue with teeth marks. Treatment includes herbs that tonify spleen yang, such as dried ginger (gan jiang), as well as moxibustion to points on the abdomen.

STOMACH SYNDROMES

All the stomach's functions involve breaking down food, so stomach disorders typically include digestive disturbances. Since the stomach and spleen are intimately related in a yin/yang polarity, imbalances in one organ often affect the other.

Stomach Fire: This syndrome of internal excess heat is characterized by a burning pain in the upper abdominal area, excessive hunger even after eating, thirst, bad breath, canker sores in the mouth, pain and bleeding in the gums, nausea, vomiting, red tongue with a thick, dry yellow coat, and a strong, rapid pulse. Some parallel Western diagnoses might be gastric ulcer or stomatitis, and treatment involves herbs that clear stomach fire, such as *Coptis* (huang lian).

Food Stagnation: This excess syndrome, usually due to overeating, can have either cold or heat signs. Symptoms include a lack of appetite, a full, bloated feeling in the stomach, nausea, vomiting, bad breath, and acid belching. Treatment of food stagnation includes herbs that move qi in the stomach, such as green tangerine peel (qing pi), along with herbs that relieve the food stagnation itself. If the person has overindulged in fatty foods, the herb of choice is hawthorn berries (shan zha); when the syndrome results from overeating of grains, barley sprouts (mai ya) are preferred.

Stomach Yin Deficiency: Symptoms of this deficiency syndrome include a lack of appetite, thirst with an inability to drink more than a few sips, dry mouth and lips, dry stools, a thin, rapid pulse, and a red tongue with no coat, especially in the center. Since the stomach yin is the source of the tongue coat, its corresponding area in the middle of the tongue appears especially peeled. This syndrome can match a Western diagnosis of chronic gastric ulcer or chronic gastritis. The herbal treatment focuses on tonifying stomach yin with herbs such as *Dendrobium* (shi hu) and *Ophiopogon* (mai men dong).

Stomach Deficient and Cold: A pattern of deficiency typically involving the spleen, it has symptoms of "dirty water stagnation": When the person moves, it is possible to hear liquids splashing. Other symptoms of this pattern are dull pains in the stomach area that are relieved by pressure and warmth, excessive sputum in the mouth, fatigue, bloating, and diarrhea. The pulse is slow, weak, slippery, and deficient, while the tongue is pale with a greasy white coat. This pattern of deficiency could possibly correspond to a Western diagnosis of food allergies, infection with the *Candida* organism, or chronic gastroenteritis. Moxibus-

Tonics made from ginseng are useful in the treatment of certain cold conditions.

tion to points on the abdomen is quite helpful in treating a cold disorder such as this. Herbal therapy includes use of herbs that are warming to the stomach such as ginger (gan jiang), tonics such as ginseng (ren shen), and dampness-draining herbs such as *Poria* (fu ling).

GALLBLADDER SYNDROMES

The gallbladder is related to the liver, both in a yin/yang relationship and physical proximity. The liver produces bile, while the gallbladder stores and secretes it. Since a strong gallbladder helps a person be assertive and decisive, imbalances in the organ can lead to indecision and timidity.

Gallbladder Damp Heat: This syndrome is described in the section on liver syndromes under "Liver and Gallbladder Damp Heat" (see page 96).

Phlegm Confusing the Gallbladder: When the gallbladder is weak and under the influence of dampness, this syndrome can develop. Its symptoms are dizziness, blurry vision, nausea, being easily startled, indecisiveness, frightening dreams, vomiting with a bitter taste, dull pain or distention in the rib area, a pale, puffy tongue with a greasy white coating, and a slippery, wiry pulse. Corresponding Western conditions might include emotional or psychological disorders, hypertension (especially in people who are overweight), and menopausal symptoms. Treatment for this syndrome includes herbal formulas that calm the spirit and clear phlegm from the gallbladder, such as Gallbladder Warming Decoction (Wen Dan Tang).

Urinary Bladder Syndromes

The urinary bladder performs the functions of receiving waste water from the kidneys and excreting it from the body. It is paired in a yin/yang relationship with the kidneys, so a deficiency in the urinary bladder is typically related to a deficiency in the kidneys. The kidneys have no excess syndromes, so any excess pattern in the urinary tract is diagnosed as a urinary bladder disharmony.

Urinary Bladder Damp Heat: This excess pattern has symptoms of pain and distention in the lower abdomen, frequent urination that is burning and produces dark urine, possible stones or blood in the urine, low back pain, and a rapid, slippery pulse. The tongue is red with a thick, greasy yellow coating, especially in the back area of the tongue, which corresponds to the lower burner. Some possible corresponding Western diagnoses are urinary tract infection, urinary tract stones, or prostate disorders. The treatment principle is to clear lower burner damp heat with herbs such as *Dianthus* (qu mai), *Phellodendron* (huang bai), and *Andrographis* (chuan xin lian).

Urinary Bladder Deficient and Cold: If the kidney qi or yang is depleted, this deficiency syndrome can occur in the bladder. Symptoms are frequent urination that is clear and copious, occasional difficulty in urinating, inability to hold in the urine, bed-wetting, feelings of cold and pain in the lower abdomen or lower back, a deep, weak pulse, and a pale, moist, puffy tongue with a thin white coat. It can be diagnosed as a chronic urinary tract infection or prostate disorder, and treatment involves moxibustion on the lower abdomen. Herbal therapy focuses on tonifying kidney yang with herbs such as *Rehmannia* (shu di huang), *Aconite* (fu zi), and cinnamon bark (rou gui).

CHAPTER 7:
Diagnosis in
Traditional Chinese Medicine

精

Diagnosis in traditional Chinese medicine may appear to be simply a grouping of symptoms, but the elegance of Chinese medicine is that a diagnosis automatically indicates a treatment strategy. For example, a woman experiencing menopause may have hot flashes, night sweats, thirst, and irritability; this group of symptoms leads to a diagnosis of kidney yin deficiency with heat. This diagnosis immediately points to the indicated therapy: Tonify kidney yin and clear deficiency heat. Since standard formulas are available for this pattern, such as Rehmannia Teapills, an accurate diagnosis enables a practitioner to prescribe a treatment that has been proved safe and effective for thousands of years.

A practitioner can obtain all of the information needed to diagnose disease through inquiry and external observation. The four basic categories of diagnostic observation are looking, listening and smelling, asking, and touching. Simply by employing these four areas of investigation, traditional practitioners can accurately assess physical and emotional imbalances of the internal organs and reestablish harmony. It is important to remember that diagnostic indicators are always viewed holistically—that is, in total and in relation to the whole person. For example, fatigue is a symptom of qi or blood deficiency, but fatigue is also a symptom in a case of wind cold. If a person with wind cold was mistakenly diagnosed with qi deficiency, he might be given ginseng, a strong tonic that would make the symptoms much worse. A careful practitioner would note that the person's pulse was strong and float-

Chinese Healing Secrets

ing, a sign of wind cold, while a person with qi deficiency would have a deep and weak pulse. While it is necessary to learn the individual diagnostic patterns, it is crucial to remember that any sign or symptom must be viewed in relation to the whole person.

LOOKING

THE FACE

An experienced practitioner often develops an initial idea of a patient's health just by observing him or her walking into the office. Inspecting the quality of the spirit (shen) is an important aspect of this first impression, since the shen gives a good indication of the overall vitality of a person. The shen especially shows in the eyes: An ancient maxim states, "If there is shen, there is life." A person with healthy shen has a gleam or sparkle of life in the eyes. The face is bright with some color, breathing is regular, and movements and speech are normal and logical. A person with unhealthy spirit has dim eyes with a vacant look. The face is dull with no shine; breathing is slow, weak, or irregular; movements appear abnormal or unusual; and speech is illogical or the voice is at an inappropriate volume.

By observing the patient's face, the practitioner can detect signs of disharmony.

Changes in facial skin color can provide the traditional Chinese medicine practitioner with a number of diagnostic clues. A bright (shiny), white face can indicate deficiency of qi or a cold condition, while a dull, pale face with no shine is a sign of blood deficiency. Redness in the face indicates heat: If the entire face is red, it is a sign of excess heat, while red cheeks alone are a sign of deficiency heat. A bright yellow skin tone can indicate damp heat, while pale yellow is a sign of damp cold due to deficiency. Finally, areas of black usually indicate kidney deficiency. The location of color on the face also has diagnostic significance as in the example of kidney deficiency: The black appears below the eyes and is often seen in people who don't get enough sleep or push themselves too hard, both practices that deplete the kidneys of qi, yin, and yang. Another example of the importance of the location of color is when it appears on the tip of the nose, an area affected by the spleen. Alcoholics often have redness in this area due to damp heat in the spleen caused by the heat generated in that organ by alcohol.

THE BODY

A lot of information can also be accumulated by looking at the overall physique. Overweight people have a tendency toward dampness or phlegm, while thin people are inclined to be yin deficient. A person with internal heat may be scantily clad in the winter, while a person with internal cold might wear a sweater in the summer. Somebody who is active and energetic tends to experience yang syndromes, while yin syndromes are more common in quiet, sedentary people. Faded, sparse, and dry hair indicates weak kidney qi or blood, while lustrous, thick, and shiny hair is a sign of strong kidney qi and sufficient blood. Finally, the lips can tell a lot about the condition of the body. Bright red lips can indicate heat, pale lips can be a sign of qi or blood deficiency, and blue lips can be due to cold or blood stagnation. Dry and cracked lips are a sign of depleted body fluids, and twitching lips are an indication of liver wind.

THE TONGUE

The most important and richest source of visual diagnostic information is the tongue. Entire books have been written to illustrate the amount of information that can be garnered simply by carefully observing the tongue. The surface of the tongue is divided into areas that correspond to the organs. The tip of the tongue corresponds to the heart, while the entire front area applies to the lungs. The middle area reflects the condition of the stomach and spleen, while the sides of the tongue are related to the liver and gallbladder. Finally, the back of the tongue corresponds to the lower burner, which includes the kidneys, the urinary bladder, and the large intestine. These assigned areas reveal a wealth of information, and they repeatedly prove accurate when applied to clinical practice.

The colors of the tongue body and coating also enhance the clinical picture. When the body of the tongue is much redder than normal, it is a sign of excess heat, while a slightly redder tongue body is a sign of deficiency heat. A pale tongue body indicates a syndrome of deficiency or cold. A purple tongue can indicate qi or blood stagnation, while a blue-tinged tongue indicates stagnation and severe deficiency of qi and blood. The consistency and shape of the tongue are also significant. A puffy tongue with teeth marks on the

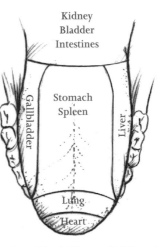

In traditional Chinese medical diagnosis, each area of the tongue surface corresponds to a particular organ.

sides is seen in a person with deficient qi, while a puffy tongue that appears wet indicates deficient yang. A shriveled, atrophied tongue is seen in deficient conditions; this sign appears sometimes in cancer patients. Finally, cracking in the tongue body occurs when body fluids have been depleted due to heat or yin deficiency.

The movements of the tongue also tell their own story. When the tongue shakes, it is a sign of deficiency or liver wind. (Of course, it can also indicate nervousness.) When a person has difficulty sticking the tongue out, it can indicate deficient qi, blood, or yin. When the tongue is turned to one side, as in stroke patients, it is a sign of internal wind or phlegm blocking the meridians. Finally, a person who leaves his tongue out, or whose tongue moves in and out, has heat in the heart.

Another important aspect of diagnosis through observation of the tongue is the appearance of the coating on the tongue. In a healthy person, the coating is thin, moist, and white. A change in the color or distribution of the coating indicates some sort of pathologic process occurring in the internal organs; for example, if there is heat in the stomach, that area of the tongue will have a yellow coating. A thick coating is related to excess conditions, while a thin coating is seen in deficiency. With yin deficiency, there is little or no coating, since the tongue coating is created by the stomach yin. An excessively moist coating is a sign of excess fluids and occurs when yang is insufficient to transform fluids (in other words, if yang is weak, fluids accumulate). A dry coating indicates fluid deficiency or dehydration; a greasy coating indicates dampness; and a patchy coating occurs when phlegm blocks the acupuncture meridians.

The color of the tongue coating can tell a lot about the nature and progress of a disease. Often, an acupuncturist requests that patients avoid brushing the tongue before an office visit, since it can take a few hours for the coating to reappear. Similarly, foods that discolor the tongue should also be avoided before an appointment, since they can make it difficult or impossible for a practitioner to read the true coating color. Although a white tongue coating is normal, it can also appear in external conditions, as well as conditions of cold or deficiency. A yellow tongue coating is always a sign of heat; as the heat increases, the intensity of the color also increases. A gray or black tongue coating can appear in conditions of extreme heat or cold, depending on the other symptoms. The progress of a disease can actually be monitored by observing the tongue over the course of an illness. A person with a high fever might have a thick yellow coating; as the fever subsides, the coating becomes more white as the excess heat leaves the body.

The practitioner checks various aspects of the patient's tongue, including the color and quality of its coating.

There are actually many more sophisticated visual diagnostic cues, but they are beyond the scope of this book. However, the above descriptions illustrate that a wealth of information is available to the observant practitioner before hearing a single word of complaint from a patient.

LISTENING AND SMELLING

Listening and smelling are two additional ways that the practitioner can garner information about a patient. The two diagnostic tools are grouped together because the same Chinese word is used for both of them. In this diagnostic area, the practitioner listens to the various sounds emanating from the patient and pays attention to any unusual smells. A wealth of information can be gleaned from these perceptions, and they give the physician some clues to pursue later on during the initial interview.

LISTENING

Speaking: A person under attack by an external pathogen speaks softly at first, with the voice gradually becoming louder. With an internal deficiency, the voice gets softer over time due to a lack of energy. People with cold syndromes tend to be quiet, while heat syndromes are associated with excessive talking. It is the nature of cold to slow functions and movement, while heat speeds them up. A person with an excess condition tends to have a loud, strong voice, while a soft, weak voice is associated with deficiency patterns. Repeated sighing is often a sign of liver qi stagnation; it is an attempt by the body to release pent-up emotion while expanding the chest muscles that tighten due to the stagnation.

Important diagnostic techniques for the traditional practitioner include looking, listening and smelling, asking, and touching.

Breathing: Weak and shallow breathing that is difficult to hear is associated with deficiency, especially of the lungs and kidneys. Loud and heavy breathing indicates an excess condition that constricts the air passages. The source of asthmatic wheezing can also be differentiated by its sounds. In a deficiency pattern, the sound is soft and the patient experiences difficulty inhaling due to the kidneys' inability to "grasp the qi." In a lung excess syndrome, the wheezing is coarse and loud and the patient has difficulty exhaling. A loud cough is a sign of excess, while a weak, slow cough is due to deficiency. A dry, hacking sound can indicate dryness or yin deficiency, while gurgling sounds are a sign of phlegm.

Gastrointestinal Signs: Vomiting due to an excess condition is loud and strong, while a deficiency condition causes vomiting that is weak and painful. Hiccups are known as "rebellious stomach qi" in traditional Chinese diagnosis. If they are due to excess, the sound is loud and short, while deficiency hiccups have a weak sound and last longer. If hiccups show up in an illness after a few days, it is an indication of a collapse of stomach qi. Loud belching is a sign of excess; if there is heat, a sour smell accompanies the belching. Deficiency belching has a softer sound with no sour smell.

SMELLING

In general, strong smells are due to heat, while a lack of aroma is a sign of cold. This applies to the breath, urine, stools, vomit, sweat, and any discharges. Some specific smells are linked to organs; for example, a sweet smell is linked to the spleen, a urine-like smell is associated with a kidney problem, and a smell like rotten apples is a sign of diabetes ("wasting and thirsting syndrome").

ASKING

This is an exceptionally important aspect of diagnosis, for Western as well as traditional Chinese practitioners. When interviewing the patient, the traditional Chinese practitioner accumulates enough information to formulate a diagnosis based on the condition of the internal organs, pernicious influences, and vital substances. The traditional Chinese practitioner also delves further into information that he or she uncovered while "looking, listening, and smelling." In addition, the practitioner attempts to get an accurate picture of the person's past medical history, lifestyle, and present area of complaint, gradually building a complete diagnostic picture.

CHILLS AND FEVER

It is important to remember that these terms refer more to the patient's perceptions of cold or heat, rather than an actual elevated body temperature or shivering. Chills and fever that occur simultaneously indicate an external condition: If the chills are worse than the fever, the condition is wind cold; if the fever is worse than the chills, it is wind heat. In either case, if the fever persists after the chills disappear, it is a sign that the condition has penetrated to the interior of the body. If the fever persists and is accompanied by sweating, thirst, and constipation, the interior heat has penetrated to the stomach and intestines, which is an even deeper level. A chronic low-grade fever can occur after an illness accompanied by a fever has "burned out the yin." This sort of fever can also be a sign of qi deficiency associated with a collapse of the body's immune system.

Feeling cold can be a symptom of either wind cold or yang deficiency. In wind cold, it can be difficult for a person to get warm, even when he or she is bundled up in warm clothes. Wind cold is an acute ailment of short duration, while yang deficiency is a long-term, chronic condition.

PERSPIRATION

Perspiration is regulated through the opening and closing of the pores, a function of the defensive qi (wei qi). When qi or yang deficiency occurs, the pores remain open due to weakness, and the person experiences spontaneous sweating during the day. This can occur even if the person has not become overheated. Sensations of heat in the evening with night sweats are considered a sign of yin deficiency. This condition is called "stealing sweats" because it steals fluids from the body like a thief in the night. In an external disorder, perspiration is an important indicator of the final diagnosis: With wind heat, the person perspires, while with wind cold, the pores are closed from cold, causing a lack of sweating. If sweating occurs with an external condition, and the person feels better afterward, it is a sign that the body has successfully expelled the pathogen. If sweating doesn't break the fever or make the person feel better, the pathogen is successfully fighting against the wei qi.

HEAD AND BODY

Headaches that have an acute onset with severe pain are usually due to an external pernicious influence, such as wind cold or wind heat. Milder, more chronic headache pain suggests an internal influence such as qi or blood deficiency. Severe, intermittent pain is likely due to liver fire, which rises

The head provides important diagnostic clues as well as acupuncture points useful in treating a variety of conditions.

up to the head, often from an outburst of anger. The location of the headache also has clinical significance, since it helps the physician select herbs and acupuncture meridians that run through the area of pain. For example, a frontal headache is considered a disorder of the stomach meridian. Treatment involves needling acupuncture points on that meridian and prescribing herbs with an affinity for that area of the body. Pain at the top or sides of the head is related to the liver and gallbladder, while pain at the back of the head is related to the bladder meridian.

Dizziness is another important diagnostic aspect associated with the head. If dizziness is due to qi deficiency, the symptoms are mild and get worse when the person is tired. Blood deficiency dizziness is also mild and gets worse when the person stands up suddenly. Dizziness from dampness is associated with a heavy feeling, which patients often describe as a "wet blanket wrapped around the head." Liver fire can create a severe form of dizziness in which the person loses balance as if on a rolling ship. If the head itself is shaking, it is a sign of internal wind moving.

Since many people turn to traditional Chinese medicine for the treatment of pain, this is often the first symptom mentioned to a practitioner. The practitioner can accumulate an abundance of information by asking about the location, severity, frequency, and causes of pain in the patient's body. Pain that comes and goes is due to wind or qi stagnation, while pain in a fixed location is a result of cold or blood stagnation. If pressure relieves the pain, it is a deficient type; pressure always makes excess type pain feel worse. Pain in specific areas of the body can also serve as a sign of problems in an internal organ. For example, pain in the rib area is a symptom of stagnation in the liver and gallbladder. Lower back pain is a cardinal sign of kidney deficiency: Since it is due to depletion, it gets worse after exertion. When low back pain is due to cold and dampness, a stagnant condition, it gets worse after rest.

EARS AND EYES

Since the kidneys open up into the ears, poor hearing or deafness is usually from kidney deficiency. Sudden deafness is usually due to heat and fire rising up to the ears, which is an excess condition. Similarly, ringing in the ears (tinnitus) is a sign of an excess condition if it comes on suddenly as a loud, high sound. Most often this is a condition of liver yang rising up to the head. Development of tinnitus over a long time is a sign of depletion of the kidneys. One diagnostic test is to press on the ears. If the sound gets stronger, it is due to excess; if it gets weaker, it is due to deficiency.

The eyes can also tell a lot about the patient. As previously mentioned, a practitioner looks into the eyes to assess the state of a person's shen (spirit) and thus acquire a general picture of the overall vitality and the potential for healing. Pain in the eyes can be due to liver fire or wind heat, while dry eyes can be caused by blood deficiency. Poor vision in general is associated with kidney jing or liver blood deficiency, as is night blindness. Itching in the eyes is a symptom of external wind or blood deficiency. Abnormal eye movement is a sign of internal wind.

STOOLS AND URINE

The stools and urine are important sources of information but may be signs overlooked by the patient. Stools that are sticky or cause burning with a strong smell are a sign of heat, while watery diarrhea with little smell is a sign of deficiency or cold. Damp heat causes frequent urges to defecate, but only a small amount is expelled each time. Stools that are watery with undigested food indicate spleen yang deficiency; if the same symptoms occur early in the morning ("cock's crow diarrhea"), it is due to kidney yang deficiency.

When constipation occurs, other diagnostic signs must be taken into account. If constipation accompanies dark urine, bad breath, and a yellow tongue coat, heat is the cause. Qi stagnation is the cause if the constipation occurs when the person is upset; qi deficiency is implicated if a person feels fatigued after a bowel movement. In blood or yin deficiency, the stools are exceptionally dry, making them difficult to pass.

Frequent passing of clear urine indicates kidney deficiency; if the urine is concentrated (dark yellow), it is a sign of heat. Bed-wetting can also occur in kidney deficiency; in children, the cause of the bed-wetting is usually emotional. Lack of urination can arise from very deficient kidneys or occur due to severe heat, blood stagnation, or a stone. Whatever its cause, lack of urination is a life-threatening condition, since the body can quickly become overwhelmed by its own toxins. In general, pale urine is a sign of cold, dark urine is a sign of heat, and cloudy urine is a sign of dampness. Sharp pain or blood in the urine can result from a stone or heat in the urinary bladder. Blood without pain could be a sign of cancer.

THIRST, APPETITE, AND TASTE

No desire for fluids at all is a sign of excess cold, while a desire for small amounts of hot liquids can indicate deficiency cold from yang depletion. A craving for large amounts of water is a sign of excess heat. If a person has a dry mouth and wants small amounts of water, it is a sign of deficiency heat due to depleted yin. If dampness is present, a person may want to drink but is unable to do so and may even vomit small amounts of water.

A person with an excessively strong appetite may have stomach heat; he or she might even eat a lot but remain thin. A person who has an appetite but no desire to eat could have stomach yin deficiency. In this case, the deficiency heat causes a false appetite, but the deficiency in stomach yin itself prevents true hunger. On the other hand, a complete lack of appetite indicates spleen qi deficiency; when the person does eat, he or she often feels bloated or tired afterward. When the appetite is low and the person has an aversion to oily foods, the cause could be damp heat in the liver and gallbladder.

Another set of diagnostic indicators unique to Chinese medicine is the presence of various tastes in the mouth. For example, a bitter taste in the mouth indicates heat, usually in the heart, liver, or gallbladder. A sweet taste can occur with damp heat in the spleen, and a salty taste can arise from a deficiency in the kidneys. A sour taste is associated with heat in the liver or food stagnation in the stomach, while a complete lack of taste can occur with spleen qi deficiency.

SLEEP

A restful night's sleep depends on a healthy balance of yin and yang. The yin and blood are the aspects of the heart that provide a solid foundation for the mind and spirit. If yin and blood are deficient, yang will be out of control. Yang is fire and activity and is kept within normal ranges by cool and calm yin. When yin is deficient, it can't control yang, and too much heat and activity results, producing such symptoms as restlessness and insomnia. On the other hand, if qi or yang is insufficient, the person experiences an overabundance of yin, leading to fatigue and excessive sleepiness. A person who has difficulty falling asleep but then sleeps soundly may have a deficiency of heart blood. Difficulty staying asleep can be a sign of deficient heart yin: The deficiency heat disturbs sleep. Insomnia that is accompanied by a bitter taste in the mouth and angry dreams is associated with liver fire, while sleeplessness due to irritability and sexual dreams can be a result of heat due to kidney yin deficiency. A person who wakes up easily, is forgetful, and experiences heart palpitations can have a pattern of insufficient heart blood and spleen qi. In children, crying at night can often be due to heat in the heart or liver.

A practitioner also attempts to determine whether a person gets too much sleep, since this could be due to qi or yang deficiency. If the person claims his whole body feels heavy, especially when the weather is rainy, the excessive sleep is caused by dampness.

LIFESTYLE AND MEDICAL HISTORY

Many imbalances are due to the patient's lifestyle. It is very difficult to treat a case of cold dampness in the spleen successfully in a person who eats a quart of ice cream every day—no matter how much ginseng and ginger the person consumes. Ice cream is classified as a cold, damp food. On the other hand, the same person can assist the healing process by consuming hot soups containing ginger root and pepper. Foods are also strong medicines with their own hot or cold energies, and selecting the proper foods for a given body type or disease pattern is an important part of the healing process. Similarly, a person who walks around barefoot in the winter might complain about frequent colds. This per-

Foods have their own medicinal properties and can therefore affect health. Hot soups containing ginseng and ginger, for example, can aid healing in a person suffering from a case of cold dampness.

son would be better off dressing in warm clothing, rather than trying to stimulate the immune system.

A complete medical history is just as important in traditional Chinese medicine as it is in Western medicine. Important clues might be uncovered that could shed light on the cause of current problems. It's important to note the use of any prescription medication, since a patient's symptoms could be due to side effects of these medications.

GYNECOLOGIC SIGNS AND SYMPTOMS

A female patient is always asked about her menstrual cycle, since it can provide abundant information about the condition of the internal organs and vital substances. A cycle that is longer than normal might be a sign of blood deficiency or cold stagnation, while a short cycle can occur with heat. A scanty menstrual flow with light-colored blood is associated with deficiency of qi and blood, while a strong flow with dark color can be a sign of excess heat. Cramping before the menstrual flow is a symptom of excess, while cramping after the flow begins is a sign of deficiency. Blood clots with sharp pains occur with blood stagnation. If there is no cycle at all, the primary causes are qi and blood deficiency or stagnation.

TOUCHING

The art of touch in traditional Chinese medicine is highly sophisticated and includes the palpation of areas of pain and diagnostic points and the reading of the patient's pulse. For example, an area of the body that feels hot to the touch is experiencing a heat condition, while a place that is cold to the touch is under the influence of cold or dampness. Tumors or swellings that are hard with a well-defined border are

Chinese Healing Secrets

due to blood stagnation, while soft nodules with an indistinct border are a result of qi or phlegm stagnation.

Diagnostic points on each acupuncture meridian can be palpated to assess the condition of an internal organ. When there is an imbalance in the organ, the point is painful or has a flaccid feeling. For example, there are points on the back known as transporting points, each one corresponding to an internal organ. If an imbalance occurs in one of these organs, the transporting point for that organ might be tender or sore. The treatment would include needling that point in order to heal the organ that is associated with it. The Japanese have also developed a highly sophisticated system of abdominal palpation; entire books have been written on the subject.

By far, the most important form of palpation in Chinese medicine is the art of pulse diagnosis. This highly sophisticated system provides abundant information about the entire body, and it can easily take an entire lifetime to become truly proficient in this ancient diagnostic method. In an ideal situation, the pulse is taken in the morning while the person is still calm and rested. In actuality, however, the procedure usually takes place in the clinic during the initial interview. It is important to let patients who have just arrived rest for a while to allow the pulses to settle down. Otherwise, it would be easy to mistake a rapid pulse for a heat condition when it is actually due to the person's hurrying to make the appointment. This is one situation when sitting in the waiting room is to the patient's advantage!

Although the pulse can be felt in a number of locations, the primary location is at the radial artery in the wrist. Each wrist has three positions that correspond to different organs. The left wrist corresponds to the heart, liver, and kidney yin. The right wrist gives information about the lungs, spleen, and kidney yang. These six positions are also felt at three different depths: deep, middle, and superficial. In addition to the information that can be gleaned from these 18 locations, the experienced practitioner can identify 28 different types of pulses. It's not hard to understand why it takes a lifetime of practice to become truly proficient at pulse-taking.

A normal pulse is strongest at the middle depth. In patterns of deficiency, the pulse is only pal-

The traditional Chinese medical practitioner will take the pulse at three different positions on both of the patient's wrists. Each position on each wrist corresponds to a specific organ.

pable at the deepest levels. A person fighting off a cold will have a strong pulse at the superficial level due to the defensive qi rushing to the surface of the body. This "floating" pulse is fairly easy for a beginner to identify, and it can be very useful clinically. Many times, this pulse appears a couple of days before a person experiences any cold symptoms, making it possible to practice early intervention. Since a rapid

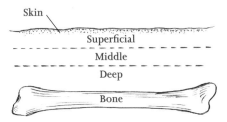

In addition to the three pulse positions on each wrist, there are three different depths—superficial, middle, and deep—at which the pulse can be felt.

pulse is a sign of heat and a slow pulse is a sign of cold, a floating, rapid pulse occurs if the condition is a case of wind heat. In this case, the pulse is also strong, since wind heat is an excess condition. A weak pulse, on the other hand, indicates a deficient condition. For example, a person with kidney yang deficiency has a deep, weak pulse, especially in the area on the right wrist that corresponds to kidney yang.

Since learning the pulses requires hands-on experience, a detailed description is beyond the scope of this book. In a clinical setting, however, students are trained to discern the following types of pulses: floating, sinking, slow, fast, empty, full, wiry, slippery, flooding, hollow, leather, soggy, hidden, confined, moderate, choppy, knotted, intermittent, hurried, spinning bean, tight, sick, scattered, small, minute, short, long, and frail. Each one of these pulses is associated with a variety of imbalances, and an experienced practitioner can learn an enormous amount of information from the pulse alone. In clinical practice, however, the physician

Traditional Chinese medicine practitioners are trained to detect more than two dozen different kinds of pulses in order to aid in the diagnosis of a variety of imbalances.

always combines the pulse information with the whole picture derived from looking, listening, smelling, and asking. Through this process, traditional Chinese practitioners are able to accurately diagnose the patterns of imbalance in their patients without the help of laboratory tests or expensive diagnostic equipment.

CHAPTER 8:
Treatments in
Traditional Chinese Medicine

肝

Once practitioners of traditional Chinese medicine make a diagnosis, they have the following options available to treat their patients: acupuncture, herbal medicine, moxibustion, cupping, exercise therapy, massage techniques, and dietary therapy. The most common therapeutic modalities are acupuncture and herbal medicine, which have such a wide range of applications, they are appropriate for most conditions. Moxibustion (the application of heat to acupuncture points or injured areas) is also widely used, while cupping (the application of suction cups to remove stagnation from an area) is often employed as an adjunct therapy for pain and stagnation. A traditional massage technique known as tui na has a profound effect on the musculoskeletal system. The Chinese also practice sophisticated forms of exercise, or movement, therapy known as qi gong and tai qi, which direct healing qi to specific areas of the body. Finally, dietary therapy is an important aspect of all healing systems, and Chinese medicine is no exception. Foods are grouped according to the organ systems they affect and whether they are hot or cold, damp or dry, yin or yang. Practitioners often advise patients about which foods to eat and which to avoid for their particular imbalance.

ACUPUNCTURE

The practice of acupuncture is based on the flow of qi, or vital energy, through pathways in the body known as channels, or meridians. Twelve regular meridians correspond to each of the six yin and six yang organs—the spleen meridian to the spleen organ, the large intestine meridian to the large intestine organ, and so on. Eight extra meridians are also used in acupuncture therapy (see page 22 for more information on meridians). Disharmony in an organ often shows up in its corresponding meridian: A person experiencing a heart attack may also have a sensation of pain and numbness that travels down the arm into the little finger, closely following the path of the heart meridian. Practitioners palpate a diagnostic point on the corresponding meridian to

assess the health of its related organ. In other cases, the meridians themselves are treated. A practitioner might treat a sore shoulder by increasing the flow of qi and blood through the large intestine, lung, and triple burner meridians. The organs related to these meridians may be completely healthy; these meridians are selected because they pass through the injured shoulder area.

A practitioner may treat a meridian because it actually passes through the area of injury or discomfort.

Although they flow deep within the body, each meridian has specific points that can be accessed from the surface of the body. There are 361 such acupuncture points on the meridians, as well as numerous "extraordinary" points that may or may not be located on a regular channel. In addition, a full set of points on the ears represent all the organs in the body and can be used to treat a wide variety of medical conditions. Use of these points is known as auriculotherapy. Acupuncture points can be stimulated by means of pressure, heat, or needling. Each point has a specific set of functions. Some of these functions have local effects, while some are systemic (affecting the body's systems as a whole). For example, the stomach meridian consists of 45 points, stretching from the head to the toes. A point just below the knee known as Dubi, or Stomach 35, is used almost exclusively for knee pain (a local effect), while the point just three inches below it, known as Zusanli (Stomach 36), has a systemic function. One of the most important points in acupuncture, Zusanli is used to treat stomach pain, vomiting, indigestion, diarrhea, constipation, dizziness, fatigue, and low immunity. Needling it often relieves stomach pain immediately. Modern research has confirmed that applying moxa or needles to this point actually raises the white blood cell count (white blood cells fight disease-causing organisms that invade the body).

As the chapter "The History of Traditional Chinese Medicine" explains, acupuncture has been practiced since ancient times with needles made from stone, wood, ivory, or bone. Modern practitioners use surgical-quality stainless steel needles with a handle wound with wire for a better grip. Some needles are plated with silver, gold, or copper to achieve special effects

Acupuncture points that are near each other may be used for very different conditions. Needling a point about three inches below the knee relieves stomach pain. Needling a point just below the knee treats knee pain.

from the treatment, such as tonification or sedation, but the majority of needles are pure steel. In the past, needles were placed in an autoclave, a device used to sterilize dental and surgical tools, after each use. However, with the increase in prevalence of hepatitis and AIDS/HIV, most practi-

DISORDERS OF THE MOUTH

- Toothache and postextraction pain
- Gingivitis
- Acute and chronic pharyngitis

GASTROINTESTINAL DISORDERS

- Spasms of esophagus and cardia
- Hiccups
- Gastroptosis
- Acute and chronic gastritis
- Gastric hyperacidity
- Chronic duodenal ulcer (pain relief)
- Acute duodenal ulcer (without complications)
- Acute and chronic colitis
- Acute bacillary dysentery
- Constipation
- Diarrhea
- Paralytic ileus

NEUROLOGIC AND MUSCULOSKELETAL DISORDERS

- Headache and migraine
- Trigeminal neuralgia
- Facial palsy (early stage)
- Pareses following a stroke
- Peripheral neuropathies
- Sequelae of early-stage poliomyelitis
- Ménière disease
- Neurogenic bladder dysfunction
- Nocturnal enuresis
- Intercostal neuralgia
- Cervicobrachial syndrome
- Frozen shoulder or tennis elbow
- Sciatica
- Low back pain
- Osteoarthritis

tioners in the West now use presterilized disposable needles to ensure absolute safety. The needles are used only once and then discarded as medical waste, which gives peace of mind to the patients, practitioners, and insurance companies.

Research in China and Japan with electrical conductivity has confirmed the tangible existence of the acupuncture points (in fact, some practitioners use "point locators" to find the exact location of an acupuncture point based on the change in electrical conductivity at the site of the point), and double-blind studies have shown acupuncture is safe and effective in treating a wide range of diseases. The World Health Organization (WHO) has compiled a list of ailments for which acupuncture treatment is effective (see pages 130–131). Of course, acupuncture is especially well known for its treatment of pain; it is so effective for pain relief, it is even used as a substitute for anesthesia in some surgical procedures in Chinese hospitals!

THE PRINCIPLE OF ACUPUNCTURE

Acupuncture treatment works on the principle that health is characterized by a smooth flow of qi and blood through the meridians and organs. When qi and blood become stagnant, pain occurs. If too much qi and blood are in a certain area, a syndrome of heat and excess can occur; too little qi and blood in an area results in a deficiency syndrome. During an acupuncture treatment, the body undergoes a normalizing process. Areas with too much qi and blood transfer these vital substances to areas that are deficient, and vice versa. The end result is a kind of homeostasis in which the body's innate wisdom brings about a self-regulatory effect. For example, the same acupuncture point can be used to treat either high or low blood pressure; similarly, another point is needled to treat both a rapid or slow heartbeat. This is one of the reasons acupuncture rarely causes side effects. It doesn't force the body to do anything; it only assists the body in performing its normal functions.

THE TECHNIQUE

Many people are surprised to learn that acupuncture is relatively painless. Unlike hypodermic needles, which are hollow and much larger, acupuncture needles can be as fine as a human hair. Many times, a patient is not even aware a needle has been inserted, especially when it is placed in areas with relatively few sensory nerves, such as the back. In a typical acupuncture treatment, the patient lies down, and the practitioner inserts needles in points that have the desired effect on the body. The patient senses heaviness, movement, or an "electrical" impulse that signals the "arrival of qi." After a few minutes, the patient typically feels a sense of calmness and well-being; many people fall asleep. After a period of 20 minutes to an hour, the practitioner removes the needles

How to Locate the Pressure Point "Great Pouring" (Taichong, Liver 3)

The point known as "Great Pouring" is one of the most important in acupuncture and acupressure. It is a soothing point, calming the mind and relieving spasms. It subdues excess yang or stimulates stagnant qi in the liver, which helps relieve migraines, frustration, anger, and the symptoms of premenstrual syndrome. The point is located on top of each foot, between the big toe and the toe next to it. To find the point, press down on the web between the toes, slide the finger toward the ankle, following the depression between the two bones (metatarsals). The point is located at the junction where the two bones meet. Often tender when pressed, it can provide immediate relief to the pain and irritability associated with liver imbalances.

Liv. 3

and advises the patient to avoid strenuous activity for a few hours to let the treatment settle in. Depending on the individual and the condition, one treatment might be sufficient, or the patient may need to return a number of times. Results can range from mild improvement to seemingly miraculous recovery. In almost all cases, however, the patient feels calmer and more peaceful after receiving acupuncture. Those who think acupuncture's success is merely a placebo effect or the patient's imagination should consider that acupuncture is exceptionally effective in animals. An increasing number of veterinarians specialize in acupuncture, and their results are quite dramatic.

In certain situations, acupuncture is inappropriate. It should not be performed if the patient is extremely hungry or full, intoxicated, or extremely fatigued. In these cases, the treatment may not be as effective or the person might experience dizziness or exhaustion. People with bleeding disorders such as hemophilia should also avoid acupuncture therapy, although careful application of acupressure or moxibustion is safe. A number of points should not be used during pregnancy due to their tendency to induce labor. Acupuncture is generally not used in children younger than 6 years of age.

Although acupuncture originated in China, a number of different branches of the field have evolved in other countries. Sophisticated systems have evolved in Japan and Korea, and development of new techniques has also occurred in Western countries such as France and England. Although extensive research has been conducted all over the world, two conclusions are commonly reached: First, acupuncture definitely works. Second, nobody is exactly sure how and why it works. This is certainly a testimonial to the brilliant clinicians who developed this miraculous healing practice over the past 2,000 years!

Herbal medicine is as old as humanity itself. Early human beings were hunter-gatherers whose survival depended on their knowledge of their environment. Direct experience taught them which plants were toxic, which ones imparted strength and sustained life, and which had special healing qualities. As mentioned in the chapter "The History of Traditional Chinese Medicine," these early discoveries were passed along until thousands of years and millions of human trials brought about the evolution of an incredibly sophisticated system of diagnosis and herbal medicine.

More than a million tons of herbs are used each year in China—an astonishing figure to many Westerners, who view herbal healing as a "new" form of treatment.

Thousands of medicinal substances are used in China today. Indeed, more than a million tons of herbs are used each year in China. Thirty herbs, mostly tonics, account for more than 50 percent of this figure, with licorice topping the list at 86,000 tons. This information may seem astonishing to the minds of Westerners, who see herbal medicine as a new development in healing. From a practical perspective, however, a fairly complete pharmacy stocks about 450 different individual herbs. From this collection of herbs, a clinical herbalist employs more than 250 standard formulas, each of which can be modified to fit a patient's individual pattern of disharmony.

The herbalist or practitioner combines herbs based on the diagnosis, using a traditional herbal formula as a foundation and adding other herbs specific to the individual's complaint and constitution. As the person's health improves, the nature of the imbalance changes, so the herb formula must also change. Some herbs are deleted when they are no longer needed, while others more appropriate to the changing condition are added.

CLASSIFICATION OF HERBAL MEDICINES

Herbs are classified according to whether they have a warming or cooling effect on the body. Their taste also has significance. Generally, sweet herbs tonify qi, sour herbs are astringent, bitter herbs dry damp and clear heat, acrid herbs disperse cold and stagnation, and salty herbs have a softening, purging effect. Both individual herbs and herbal formulas are organized into categories, based on diagnostic patterns. For example, if a person has deficient kidney yang, the practitioner selects herbs from the category of "herbs that tonify yang." The therapeutic categories of herbs follow:

Herbs that Release the Exterior: When the body's protective qi is repelling a pathogenic influence, the struggle occurs in the exterior layers of the body. Herbs in this category have an outward dispersing action, preventing the disease from penetrating to the interior of the body. Warm herbs of this type expel wind cold by inducing perspiration and warming the body; cool, acrid herbs are chosen to repel wind heat.

Herbs that Clear Heat: This category of cooling herbs clears all kinds of internal heat—excess heat, heat from deficiency, heat in the blood, heat with toxicity, and damp heat.

Downward Draining Herbs: These herbs treat differing degrees of constipation and are used as cathartics, purgatives, and mild lubricating laxatives.

Herbs that Drain Dampness: This category contains herbs that remove dampness in the form of edema (swelling due to fluid retention) or urinary disorders.

Herbs that Dispel Wind Dampness: Used mostly for arthritis and skin conditions, these herbs increase circulation and reduce swelling and inflammation.

Herbs that Transform Phlegm and Stop Coughing: Some of these herbs relax the cough reflex, others clear phlegm. For heat phlegm, cooling moistening expectorants are chosen; warming drying expectorants are used to treat cold phlegm.

Aromatic Herbs that Transform Dampness: If dampness overwhelms the digestive organs, these herbs penetrate the dampness with their aroma and revive the spleen.

Herbs that Relieve Food Stagnation: When food is stuck in the stomach and won't move, this category of herbs is chosen in order to move the stagnation.

Herbs that Regulate Qi: These herbs remove stagnation from the digestive system and move qi that is stuck in the liver.

Herbs that Regulate Blood: Herbs in this category are divided into those that stop bleeding and those that increase circulation and remove stagnation.

Herbs that Warm the Interior: Warming the metabolism at a deep level, these herbs dispel cold conditions and revive the digestive fire—the metabolic energy required to digest food. When it is low (as in spleen yang deficiency), digestion is weak and the person craves warm foods and liquids.

Tonifying Herbs: Divided into herbs that tonify yin, yang, qi, or blood, this is the superior category of medicines. These herbs can prevent disease rather than simply treat disease that has already appeared. Nourishing and strengthening, they can be used long-term to correct deficiencies of the vital substances (qi, blood, body fluids, essence).

How to Make a Traditional Herbal Decoction

The strongest herbal medicines are in the form of decoctions. A decoction is a concentrated herbal tea made by boiling herbs in water. Making a decoction requires some patience, and drinking one requires a tolerance for very strong tastes and aromas. To make a standard decoction:

1. Place the herbs in a pot, preferably one made of ceramic or glass. Stainless steel is an acceptable alternative, but never use iron or aluminum because they have a tendency to react chemically with the herbs. Aluminum is also a toxic heavy metal, so it should not be used for any type of food preparation.

2. Add 3 cups of cold water to the herbs. Bring the water to a boil over high heat. Reduce to medium heat and continue to boil the herbs until 1 cup of liquid remains (approximately 20 minutes).

3. Strain this liquid and set it aside. This is one dose of herbal medicine.

4. Add 2 cups of water to the previously cooked herbs (they have already absorbed water, so they need less). Boil them again until 1 cup of liquid remains.

Astringent Herbs: These herbs dry excessive secretions, such as diarrhea, excessive urination, or sweating.

Herbs that Calm the Spirit: These substances have a calming effect and are used for anxiety, insomnia, palpitations, and irritability.

Herbs that Open the Heart: Containing aromatic substances, usually resins, these herbs can revive a person's consciousness. Some are used for conditions such as angina.

Herbs that Clear Internal Wind and Tremors: These herbs treat muscle spasms, hypertension, and involuntary movements.

5. Strain this liquid and add this second dose to the first.

6. Repeat steps 4 and 5 to make a third dose. Mix the doses thoroughly so you end up with 3 cups of concentrated decoction.

7. Discard the herbs, preferably in your compost pile.

8. Take 1 cup of decoction three times a day for an acute ailment or one cup per day over three days for chronic conditions.

The reason for making three 20-minute decoctions instead of one 1-hour decoction is simple. Some of the herbs in a formula will likely contain volatile aromatic oils as their active ingredient. These volatile oils can be captured in a 20-minute boiling, but they will be lost by the end of an hour. On the other hand, it might take a full hour to fully extract the medicinal constituents in hard roots. For this reason, combine all three doses and then separate them again into three equal doses to ensure that all three doses have the same balance of constituents and flavors.

Herbs that Expel Parasites: These herbs can destroy or expel various parasites from the body.

Substances for External Application: These consist of herbs and minerals, many of them toxic if taken internally, that are applied topically for skin problems, bruises, spasms, and sprains.

Herbal formulas also are divided into the same diagnostic categories. The traditional formulas, or patent medicines, are an intricate combination of herbs chosen to address the various aspects of a disease pattern. The *chief* herb in the formula addresses the major complaint; the formula usually contains more of this particular herb than other herbs. The *deputy* herb assists the chief herb in its function, while the *assistant* herb reinforces the effects of the chief and deputy or performs a secondary function. The *envoy* directs the formula to a certain part of the body, or it harmonizes and detoxifies the other parts of the formula. For example, Ephedra Decoction is used for wind cold with wheezing, stiff neck from cold, and a lack of sweating. *Ephedra* is the chief herb, since it treats all of the main symptoms. Cinnamon twig is the deputy because it assists *Ephedra* in promoting sweating and warming the body. Apricot seed acts as the assistant by focusing on the wheezing, while licorice is the envoy because it harmonizes the actions of the other herbs and restrains the *Ephedra* from inducing too much sweating. Larger formulas may have multiple herbs that produce the different functions, depending on the desired action of the formula.

Herbs can be taken in the form of decoctions, pills, liquid extracts, powdered extracts, and syrups. Decoctions tend to be the strongest medicine, followed by concentrated liquid extracts, concentrated pow-

精 How to Make an Immune Tonic Soup

A number of tonifying herbs in Chinese medicine also strengthen the immune system, in addition to their other valuable functions. Of these, a few have a bland or slightly sweet taste, making them suitable as ingredients in soups. Incorporating medicine with food is quite a common practice in China, and it is especially useful with children or adults who don't like to take herbs in other forms.

The most commonly used tonic herbs in a soup stock are *Astragalus* root, *Codonopsis* root, *Dioscorea* yam, and lotus seed. The following simple recipe makes about two servings.

> 10 grams *Astragalus membranaceus* root (huang qi)
>
> 10 grams *Codonopsis pilosula* root (dang shen)
>
> 10 grams *Dioscorea opposita* yam (shan yao)
>
> 10 grams lotus seed (*Nelumbo nucifera*) (lian zi)

Boil the herbs in 6 cups of water until half the liquid is gone. Remove the *Astragalus* and *Codonopsis* and add some kale, carrots, potato, shiitake mushrooms, seaweed, or other vegetables in season. Continue cooking until the vegetables are soft, and remove from the heat. Mix in some miso according to taste. The yam and lotus seeds should be soft and edible at this point.

These herbal ingredients can be adapted to *any* soup recipe; simply boil them and remove after about 30 minutes. The remaining liquid can be used as stock in your favorite soup recipe.

dered extracts, and pills. All are effective, and the use of the different forms depends on the individual's personal choice. If you don't have the time to make a decoction or you don't like the taste, pills or capsules will be more effective, simply because you'll be more likely to take them. The concentrated liquid extracts tend to take effect quickly, so they are useful in cases where fast action is important, and the syrups are good for sore throats or as tonics. However, many of the more concentrated extracts are available only from a health care practitioner. In whatever form they are taken, though, accurately prescribed herbal formulas are exceptionally effective in restoring health and vitality. This ancient art of traditional herbal medicine is, without a doubt, one of China's great gifts to humanity.

MOXIBUSTION

Moxibustion, or moxa, is named after the Japanese word mokusa, meaning "burning herb." It was first recorded in medical texts during the Song Dynasty (A.D. 960), but it has most likely been in use much longer. It is an important therapy in traditional Chinese medicine; the ancient texts advise that moxa should be tried if acupuncture and herbs have failed to heal the disease. The heat from moxibustion is very penetrating, making it effective for impaired circulation, cold and damp conditions, and yang deficiency. When applied to acupuncture points specific for yang deficiency, the body absorbs the heat into its deepest levels, restoring the body's yang qi and "life-gate fire," the source of all heat and energy in the body.

For indirect moxa, the moxa wool is rolled into a cigar shape, wrapped in paper, and lighted.

Moxa is prepared from mugwort (*Artemisia vulgaris*), which is a common perennial herb. The aromatic leaves are dried and repeatedly sifted until they are fluffy.

How to Moxa the Point "Leg Three Miles" (Zusanli, Stomach 36)

The point called Zusanli, or "Leg Three Miles," was named after its legendary ability to boost the vital energy of the body, making it useful for preparing for long trips on foot. Although the point can be activated by pressure or needling, moxibustion is the preferred method when the goal is to build energy, or qi.

The point is located under the knee on both legs, approximately the width of four fingers below the bottom of the knee cap (patella), and one finger width away from the shinbone (tibia), in an outward lateral direction.

After lighting a moxa stick, hold the glowing end about an inch away from the point, maintaining as much heat as possible without discomfort. After 5 or 10 minutes on each leg, carefully extinguish the moxa in a bowl of salt or sand or with water. Never try to put it out by crushing it in an ash tray, since it will continue smoldering and be a fire hazard.

There are two heating techniques used to apply moxibustion: indirect moxa and direct moxa. In indirect moxa, the "moxa wool" is rolled into a long cigar shape and wrapped in paper. The cigar-shaped moxa stick is then lighted and held about an inch away from the desired area—an acupuncture point or other area of the body chosen by the practitioner. Indirect moxa can be used on acupuncture points to achieve a systemic, or bodywide, effect or it can be used directly at the site of a problem. For example, indirect moxa might be applied to a swollen, stiff area such as an arthritic joint. It is also appropriate to apply indirect heat to specific acupuncture points, such as Zusanli (Stomach 36) or Mingmen (Du 4), to create a systemic effect. The heat taken into these points raises the body's metabolism and immunity, so moxibus-

Chinese Healing Secrets

tion at these points can also be used in preventive health care. One ancient text declares that "one who applies moxa daily to Zusanli (Stomach 36) will be free of the one hundred diseases." Applying moxa to Stomach 36 has an energizing effect on the body, especially in regard to immune and digestive functions. Some indications for its use in Chinese medicine are to treat general weakness, anemia, indigestion, nausea, chronic fatigue, shock, allergies, and asthma. Modern research has confirmed that the immune system is stimulated when the point receives moxa.

Another type of indirect moxa involves rolling the moxa, placing it on the end of an acupuncture needle while the needle is in the body, and igniting it. The heat from the moxa travels down the handle and into the needle. The needle transfers the heat specifically to the desired point on the body.

In direct moxibustion, a small amount of herb is rolled into a cone and burned directly on the skin. This can sometimes cause a burn, so this technique is rarely performed in Western acupuncture clinics. In most cases when moxa is applied directly to the skin, some ointment is first placed on the point to avoid a burn. In other techniques, the moxa is burned on top of a slice of ginger, garlic, or aconite; this prevents a burn and also adds the therapeutic effects of those herbs to the treatment.

In all cases, moxibustion can be a very pleasant sensation, especially when the warmth spreads through areas that have pain and swelling due to cold. Indirect moxa is also easy to learn to do at home. Practitioners often show a patient the appropriate point for their condition, and the person can take a moxa stick home to perform daily treatments. Such treatment can be very empowering, since the patient then takes responsibility for his own healing.

CUPPING

Cupping is a fascinating therapy in which a special cup or jar is attached to the skin by means of suction. The suction is created by heating the air inside the cup to create a vacuum, then quickly pressing the mouth of the cup to the desired area. There are also modern cups that

In cupping, the air inside the cup is heated to create a vacuum, then the cup is quickly pressed onto the desired area.

can be applied with a suction device. Interestingly, cultures all over the world are known to use this technique, making it virtually a universal practice. In ancient times, it was done with bamboo cups or animal horns, and it was often employed to treat external conditions of the skin and muscles such as sprains and strains and drawing out pus. It is especially effective for musculoskeletal pain, often relieving the pain after a single application. The force of the suction draws stagnant blood to the surface of the body, sometimes leaving a round bruise in the shape of the cup. Since pain is caused by the stagnation of qi and blood, the goal of this therapy is to remove the stagnation, increase circulation, and allow healing to take place.

Cupping should not be used when the patient has broken skin, skin ulcers, edema, high fever, bleeding disorders, varicose veins, or convulsions. It should also not be performed on the abdomen or low back of a woman who is pregnant. Care needs to be taken to avoid burning the patient with a hot cup; using the cups with the suction device eliminates this potential problem.

The practice of qi gong is exceptionally common in China. On any given morning, parks all over the country are filled with people of all ages practicing the graceful movements of both qi gong and tai qi. While most people perform these exercises for their own benefit, a practitioner can impart healing energy to a patient's body through medical qi gong methods.

QI GONG

Qi gong (pronounced chee guhng) has been practiced in China in its various forms for thousands of years. It consists of exercises involving specific breathing practices and/or movements, with the goal of enhancing and balancing qi. The central principle involves meditating on a vital energy center known as the Dantian (pronounced dahn tyehn). Located about three inches below the navel, it is considered the root of qi in the body. By focusing on this area while moving the body, a person is able to build up a storehouse of qi and direct it to areas that need it.

Qi gong exercises have been practiced in China for thousands of years.

Qi gong has a wide variety of forms, ranging from quiet meditative exercises that bring about a sense of peace and well-being to techniques that send powerful waves of energy flowing through the body. In its medical form, qi gong is used to build immunity, treat disease, improve strength, clarify the mind, and enable a person to tap into underlying reserves of energy. The ancient Chinese physician Hua Tuo is quoted as saying "a running stream never goes bad," meaning that qi and blood will not become stagnant if proper exercise keeps them circulating. He developed a set of exercises known as "imitation of five animals boxing," which was an early form of both qi gong and tai qi. He and his followers were able to remain healthy into old age by practicing these exercises regularly.

As Chinese medicine grew more sophisticated over time, the practice of qi gong also became more focused on curing specific diseases. By the 19th century, it was used clinically for ailments such as indigestion, toothache, eye problems, headache, abdominal pain, and chronic degenerative diseases in general.

The practitioner of qi gong trains in order to master three groups of exercises: those that regulate the body, those that regulate the heart and mind, and those that regulate breathing. The purpose of these exercises is for the practitioner to learn to release muscular tension, strengthen the muscles and tendons, and circulate qi and blood to the various organs and regions of the body. Different positions are assumed, depending on the desired result, but in all cases a profound relaxation allows the muscles and organs to rest and rejuvenate. Meditating on the Dantian also allows the practitioner of qi gong to become free of distracting thoughts, bringing about a state of inner peace and heightened awareness. In medical qi gong, it is possible to direct the healing energy to specific organs and meridians. The patient can do this, and it is also possible for the physician to direct healing qi into the patient's body through his or her hands. When qi gong is combined with acupuncture treatment, the therapeutic results can be truly remarkable. For example,

Chinese Healing Secrets

this therapy can be used to help stroke victims begin to talk or walk again, sometimes after only one treatment.

Much research into the physiologic effects of qi gong has been conducted in modern-day China. Studies have shown a drastic alteration of brain wave patterns and a radical decrease in adrenaline, a hormone secreted in response to stress. Heart rate slows, blood pressure decreases, cholesterol levels can drop, and the immune system is strengthened by increased production of blood cells. Physicists studying the effects of qi gong at research institutes have actually discovered quantifiable changes during the practice of qi gong, such as the body's production of low levels of energy in the form of infrared energy, visible light, static electricity, and even ultraviolet and microwave radiation. Much more research remains to be done in this fascinating field, but one finding is certain: Qi gong is a powerful therapeutic modality capable of promoting wellness and healing disease. It stands well on its own and is also an effective adjunct to other traditional therapies.

and hands facing down in your lap, meditate on the Dantian as you inhale normally. Continue focusing on the Dantian while you exhale normally, then slowly lean forward and slide your hands out in front of you on the floor. You should be fully stretched out by the end of the exhale, not forcing either the stretch or the breathing. Gradually sit up to the original position as you inhale, continuing your meditation on the energy center. Repeat for a few minutes, then discontinue the focused meditation and sit still with your eyes closed, breathing normally.

After a qi gong session, people typically feel energized and relaxed, ready to deal with the stresses of the world in a calm and grounded manner.

THERAPEUTIC MASSAGE (TUI NA)

No healing modality could possibly be older than massage, since it is such a basic human instinct to rub a painful area. The Chinese have developed a sophisticated system of massage over a period of thousands of years that is used for numerous conditions. Going far beyond the expected applications for musculoskeletal pain, this massage technique is taught in Chinese medical schools, and specialists in the art are able to treat a wide range of diseases effectively. By working with the meridian system, practitioners are able to treat internal conditions such as hypertension, peptic ulcer, insomnia, nausea, arthritis, and constipation.

These Chinese monks are practicing the system of therapeutic massage known as tui na.

Pediatric massage is a field of specialty practiced in Chinese hospitals. It is especially effective on children younger than 5 years of age, and the younger the child, the more effective the treatment tends to be. The caress of a loving parent is the first sensation a baby experiences after birth, and recent research in the West has shown that infants who are routinely touched tend to be healthier and gain more weight. Some of the conditions treated by pediatric tui na, or massage, are diarrhea, vomiting, poor appetite, common cold, fever, bed-wetting, and crying at night. As in adult therapeutic massage, pediatric massage involves a variety of manipulations, such as pushing, spreading, kneading, pinching, and pressing. The manipulations are chosen according to the level of stimulation desired and the nature of the area massaged.

The results of Chinese therapeutic massage can often be quite dramatic, bringing about an immediate sense of healing. It is especially effective when used with other modalities, such as herbal medicine. For example, in an injury, herbs are taken internally to reduce the inflammation, swelling, and pain. In addition, a topical herb formula is combined with oil and massaged into the injured area to increase circulation and healing to the area, augmenting the systemic effect of the internal formula. This sort of three-pronged approach ensures a much faster recovery time, and it is one of the reasons that tui na practitioners are held in such high regard in China.

DIETARY THERAPY

Chinese dietary therapy is an integral part of any complete treatment plan. The earliest written record is Sun Simiao's *Prescriptions Worth a Thousand Gold*, published in A.D. 652, in which he discusses the treatment of a variety of diseases through diet. For example, his treatment for goiter included the use of seaweed and the thyroid glands from farm animals.

This early iodine and hormone replacement therapy predates Western discoveries by hundreds of years. Similarly, in A.D. 752, Wang Shou published *A Collection of Diseases*, in which he describes his treatment for diabetes. He recommended the use of pork pancreas as a treatment, predating the discovery of insulin by 1,000 years. In the absence of laboratory tests, his method of checking for sugar in the urine was ingenious: The patient was instructed to urinate on a flat brick to see if ants would show up to collect the sugar!

In the traditional system of dietary cures, foods have been organized into categories based on their innate temperature, energetics (the direction in which they move qi and how they affect qi and blood flow), and the organs they affect. For example, a person who has a wind cold condition with excessive clear mucus might be told to consume hot soup made from onions and mustard greens. The onions are warming, expel cold, and sedate excess yin. The mustard greens have similar prop-

 ## How to Make Rice Congee

The food most commonly used for therapeutic effects is congee, a rice gruel that is soothing to the stomach and exceptionally easy to digest. It is made by slowly cooking 1 part white rice in 6 parts water until the rice is the consistency of a thick soup. A crock pot works especially well for this purpose. In China, the previous day's leftovers are typically cooked into the congee in large pots. In the morning, people gather to have the congee for breakfast. As a therapy, specific ingredients can be added for their medicinal effect. For example, an elderly person who is experiencing constipation due to yang deficiency might add walnuts for their tonifying and lubricating actions. A person who is experiencing weak vision due to blood deficiency could add *Lycium* fruit for its ability to nourish the eyes.

Chinese Healing Secrets

erties, and they also help expel mucus and relieve chest congestion. Flavoring the soup with ginger and black pepper enhances the warming, expectorant action. With such a lunch, one can imagine that the person's herb formula would be much more effective. On the other hand, if the same patient decided to have salad for lunch with a cold glass of milk, the cold and damp nature of this meal would make the wind cold condition much worse. Any herbal therapy administered at this point would be much less effective, since the therapy first needs to overcome the negative effect of the food before dealing with the acute ailment. For this reason, a patient is always advised about which foods could exacerbate the imbalance and which will help restore balance.

In general, grains and beans are considered to bring stability to the body. They build blood and qi, and they establish rhythm and stability. Vegetables, which are best if eaten in season, bring vitality. Leafy greens have an affinity for the upper body, while root vegetables give strength to the middle and lower body. Fruits build fluids and purge toxins, and they tend to be cooling by nature. They should be eaten alone, or they can cause indigestion. Meats possess the full range of temperatures, and they are a simple source of blood. But they are meant to be consumed in small quantities; their overconsumption in Western countries has caused an epidemic of heart disease. Finally, dairy products are a good source of fats, but they should also be eaten in moderation. Overconsumption can result in excess dampness or mucus. A healthy diet should consist mainly of a wide variety of organically grown whole grains, beans, and vegetables; fruits and animal protein should be eaten in smaller amounts. While it is possible to have a healthy, well-balanced vegetarian diet, people who eat no animal products at all (vegans) should supplement their diet with vitamin B$_{12}$. Other general principles relating to diet appear in the chapter "Patterns of Disharmony."

A TYPICAL TREATMENT PLAN

A practitioner of traditional Chinese medicine may specialize in acupuncture only or herbal medicine only; other practitioners practice both. On its own, each therapy system can effectively treat a wide range of diseases. However, most practitioners agree that a highly effective treatment consists of a combination of acupuncture and herbal medicine.

A typical treatment plan might consist of an acupuncture treatment once a week with herbs taken between treatments. This combination of acupuncture and herbal therapy is applied often in the West, where most people must pay out of their own pockets for acupuncture treatments. In China's socialized medical system, a person might receive free acupuncture daily for two weeks as a course of treatment, take a break for a few days, and then undergo another course of treatment. But in the West, unless a patient's insurance policy covers alternative medical practices,

A clinical herbalist employs more than 250 standard formulas, each of which can be modified to suit a patient's individual pattern of disharmony.

this sort of treatment plan is simply too expensive for most people. Using herbal therapy between acupuncture treatments provides continuous treatment at a lower cost to the patient.

水 The Energetics of Foods

Chinese medicine recognizes that foods have an innate temperature that can warm or cool the body, much the same way herbs can. The food we eat can have a profound positive or negative effect on healing. For example, the condition of a person with chronic inflammation due to heat arising from yin deficiency is more likely to improve if this person eats cooling, moistening foods such as lettuce, cucumbers, and mung beans. On the other hand, if he or she eats warming, drying foods such as chicken with ginger and onions, the condition will be more difficult to resolve, even if the person is taking cooling herbs. Since they don't affect the body's interior climate, neutral foods are appropriate in most situations.

Cold

Banana	Persimmon	Clam	Kelp
Grapefruit	Tomato	Crab	Salt
Watermelon	Seaweed		

Cool

Apple	Strawberry	Radish	Tofu
Tangerine	Eggplant	Spinach	Wheat
Orange	Cucumber	Barley	Seasame oil
Pear	Lettuce	Mung bean	Peppermint

Acupuncture and herbal therapy also work in a synergistic fashion, supporting each other. In the case of a knee injury, for example, acupuncture needles are inserted at the site of injury to increase the flow of qi to the injured area. To accentuate the effect, herbs are prescribed that have a general strengthening and anti-inflammatory action. As the inflammation subsides, moxibustion and massage are added to the treatment plan. As the patient's condition further improves, qi gong

Neutral

Fig	Carrot	Shiitake	Milk
Grape	Celery	mushroom	Egg
Olive	Beet	Yam	Pork
Papaya	Corn	Green beans	Carp
Pineapple	Potato	Rice	Oysters
Plum	Sweet potato	Soybean	Honey
Peanut	Pumpkin	Beef	White sugar
Cabbage			

Warm

Cherry	Asparagus	Mutton	Fennel
Coconut	Green onion	Chicken	Basil
Guava	Leek	Mussel	Dill
Date	Onion	Shrimp	Garlic
Peach	Squash	Vinegar	Clove
Raspberry	Mustard	Wine	Nutmeg
Chestnut	greens	Coffee	Coriander
Walnut	Malt syrup	Brown sugar	Rosemary
Chive	Sweet rice	Fresh ginger	Spearmint

Hot

Soybean	Dried ginger	Black pepper	Red pepper
Cinnamon			

and tai qi exercises are added to the treatment plan to bring additional strength and qi flow to the area of healing.

There is no typical duration of treatment in traditional Chinese medicine, since each case is treated individually. A person with an acute, but simple, condition might feel completely free of illness and pain after just one acupuncture treatment, while another person with a chronic disorder might require weekly acupuncture and daily herbal medicine for a few months before the condition is rectified. In all cases, however, the practitioner chooses the treatment modality he or she believes will be most effective in view of the practitioner's experience and the individual receiving treatment.

While all the treatment methods described here are part of an ancient tradition, Chinese medicine continues to evolve. New treatment modalities have been tested and introduced, such as electroacupuncture (in which a mild electrical current is applied to the needles to provide a stronger and more continuous stimulation—a useful technique when stronger stimulation is desired, as in cases of paralysis), magnetic therapy, laser acupuncture (in which the points are stimulated with a special laser, a technique favored by people afraid of needles), and various types of healing radiation. With the wealth of knowledge from the past joining the ingenuity of the future, traditional Chinese medicine possesses a powerful set of tools for the treatment of disharmony and disease in all its forms.

CHAPTER 9:
Finding a Qualified Practitioner

Acupuncture and traditional Chinese herbal medicine have been practiced quietly in Asian communities in the United States for more than 150 years. It remained "underground" as an isolated cultural phenomenon until 1971, when interest was sparked by the experience of *The New York Times* reporter James Reston. His experience of acupuncture in China led him to write an article in which he stated, "I have seen the past, and it works."

At the time Reston's article appeared, no states had any legislation regarding acupuncture. By 1976, eight states had legalized acupuncture and six schools had been established. Twenty years later, as this book is being written, there are more than 40 schools of Oriental medicine, and 29 states and the District of Columbia have licensing laws that regulate acupuncturists. Legislation has been drafted or introduced in

In China today, patients are treated with both Western medicine and traditional Chinese medicine. Today in the United States, where the number of traditional Chinese medicine practitioners is increasing, more and more patients are also reaping the benefits of both healing systems.

12 other states. The U.S. Food and Drug Administration (FDA) estimates that between 8 and 12 million people receive acupuncture each year in the United States, and its popularity continues to increase as more peo-

ple hear of its effectiveness. No longer considered a fringe element, acupuncture has been endorsed by the American Osteopathic Association, the American Chiropractic Association, and the American Veterinary Medical Association. It has been incorporated into the substance abuse treatment programs of more than 20 hospitals in the United States and is considered so effective that drug offenders in Florida's Miami-Dade County have a choice of either receiving acupuncture treatment or going to jail. In Portland, Oregon, drug offenders in the treatment program must receive acupuncture as a condition of their probation or parole. Gradually, hospitals and conventional medical practices are also adding acupuncturists to their staff as the demand for their services continues to grow.

Before choosing a practitioner--any health practitioner-- it is important to discuss with them your needs and health problems, their treatment style and qualifications, fees for services, and similar issues.

Now that acupuncture and traditional Chinese medicine are rapidly entering the mainstream of the practice of medicine in North America, an increasing number of people are interested in finding a qualified practitioner. As with all professional services, the best way to find a practitioner is through a referral. If a trusted friend or relative has had favorable experiences with a practitioner, many people will feel safe consulting that physician. Referrals are relatively easy to come by in places such as California, where there are thousands of practitioners;

most people know somebody who has received acupuncture or herbal therapy. However, in many areas this isn't the case; it is necessary to find a practitioner without the advice of a friend or relative.

Fortunately, there are certifying agencies that establish standards that a practitioner must meet to be considered qualified. The most established is the National Certification Commission for Acupuncture and Oriental Medicine (NCCA), in Washington D.C. (see Resources on page 249). After three to four years of training, a student is qualified to sit for a licensing exam. The NCCA's extremely high standards for scholastics and clinical training become evident to any student who has been through this rigorous process. Since 1984, it has certified more than 7,000 practitioners of acupuncture and more than 1,000 practitioners of Chinese herbology. NCCA certification is used as the basis for licensure in 90 percent of the states that have set standards for the practice of acupuncture. The NCCA will provide a list of the certificate holders to anybody seeking a qualified practitioner.

A number of national acupuncture and Oriental medicine foundations also provide referrals (see Resources on page 249). The American Association of Oriental Medicine advises prospective patients of qualified practitioners in their area. For those who have access to the Internet, an excellent place to find referrals is at the Web site www.acupuncture.com. The site lists practitioners all over the world in addition to North America, and it is also a good source of interesting information about traditional Chinese medicine.

Generally, the yellow pages lists practitioners under Acupuncturists. It is well within your rights to call practitioners and ask them about their training and experience. If you have a particular condition, ask them if they have any experience in treating it. Like all professions, skill levels

Legislative Update
(as of November 1996)

JURISDICTIONS THAT LICENSE,
CERTIFY, OR REGISTER ACUPUNCTURISTS

Alaska	Maryland	Pennsylvania
California	Massachusetts	Rhode Island
Colorado	Minnesota	South Carolina
Connecticut	Montana	Texas
District of Columbia	Nevada	Utah
Florida	New Jersey	Vermont
Hawaii	New Mexico	Virginia
Iowa	New York	Washington
Louisiana	North Carolina	West Virginia
Maine	Oregon	Wisconsin

JURISDICTIONS THAT ALLOW PRACTICE THROUGH A RULING
BY THE BOARD OF MEDICAL EXAMINERS

Kansas	Michigan	Missouri

LEGISLATION IN PROGRESS

Alabama	Idaho	Ohio
Arizona	Illinois	Oklahoma
Arkansas	Michigan	Tennessee
Georgia	New Hampshire	Wyoming

vary. It is also important to work with somebody with whom you feel comfortable. In some areas, other health care professionals might provide a referral to an acupuncturist, especially if they work in a holistic group practice.

If you're seeking a qualified traditional Chinese herbalist, the NCCA also provides a list of practitioners who have passed their exam on herbal medicine. Otherwise, a good place to look is California. As of this writing, it is the only state that requires a practitioner to be proficient in herbal medicine in order to pass the state licensing exam. For this reason, schools of Oriental medicine in California have four-year programs, while most schools outside of California have three-year programs. This is rapidly changing, and some schools outside of California now offer a thorough exposure to herbal medicine. There are also many good herbalists outside of California who haven't yet taken the relatively new Herbalism exam. These practitioners can often be found by a referral from a satisfied patient.

CHAPTER 10:
Treatment of Common Ailments in Traditional Chinese Medicine

This chapter describes some common ailments that can be treated successfully with traditional Chinese medicine. Each disorder is explained in the context of possible Chinese diagnoses, and a typical treatment plan is described. Treatment might include a combination of acupuncture, herbal medicine, moxibustion, qi gong, and massage therapy, depending on the ailment. Treatment also depends on the style and training of the practitioner: Some specialize in acupuncture alone, while others rely mostly on herbs or other modalities. Still, the most common treatment plan is a combination of acupuncture and herbal medicine, and this is reflected in the sample treatment plans in this chapter. A practitioner may create an herbal formula specifically for your condition or prescribe a Chinese patent medicine. A description of common patent medicines follows this section (pages 191–248); references to these patent formulas appear in boldface type in this section.

It is very important to remember that the purpose of this section on ailments and the following section is to give an idea of how a practitioner of Chinese medicine views and treats common ailments. The information is not meant to replace qualified medical care, nor is it in any way intended to be a complete discussion of the given ailments. After consulting this book, seek the help of a qualified health care practitioner for an accurate diagnosis and treatment plan.

Allergies

Allergies occur when the body's immune system misidentifies a normally harmless substance as a threat to the body. Common allergens (substances that produce allergic reactions) are foods, pollen, animal dander, mold, insect venom, drugs, and dust mites. An inflammatory reaction takes place in an attempt to eject this substance from the system, resulting in a variety of symptoms. A traditional Chinese medical treatment for pollen allergies, or hay fever, follows.

Several Chinese patterns of disharmony may be involved in cases of allergies. In all cases, however, wind is part of the diagnosis, usually combining with another pathogenic influence in wind dampness, wind cold, or wind heat. Typical of patterns involving wind, allergy symptoms often occur without warning. In seasonal allergies, such as hay fever, the most common diagnosis is wind and dampness. This combination produces a sudden onset of symptoms: sneezing, itching eyes and throat, and a heavy sensation in the head with copious mucus. The treatment strategy is to repel the wind with herbs that are dispersing in nature, such as Japanese catnip (*Schizonepeta tenuifolia*, jing jie) and *Siler divaricata* (fang feng). Herbs that drain dampness are also employed in order to clear the nasal passages and sinuses; the major herbs for this purpose are *Angelica dahurica* (bai zhi), magnolia flower buds (xin yi hua), and *Xanthium sibiricum* (cang er zi). This combination is known as Xanthium Decoction. An appropriate patent medicine is **Bi Yan Pian**.

Typically, an underlying weakness, often a deficiency of lung and spleen qi, makes persons with allergies susceptible to allergic reactions. Lung qi is responsible for the proper function of the entire respiratory tract, including the nasal passages. Spleen qi controls the transport of fluids; when spleen qi is impaired, weakening digestive function, it can lead to an overproduction of mucus, which tends to collect in the lungs. This weakness of qi is treated with tonifying herbs that bolster lung and spleen function, such as *Codonopsis* (dang shen), *Atractylodes* (bai zhu), *Poria* (fu ling), and prepared licorice (zhi gan cao). An appropriate patent medicine for this type of deficiency is **Six Gentlemen Teapills**. This formula also contains *Pinellia* (ban xia) and aged citrus peel (chen pi), which enhance the base formula's ability to clear mucus and dry dampness. A traditional Chinese medicine practitioner may customize the formula to meet a patient's individual needs. For example, *Chrysanthemum* flowers (jua hua) and *Cassia* seeds (jue ming zi) can be added to soothe itchy eyes, and jujube dates (da zao) can be included to enhance the overall antiallergic action of the formula.

Diet plays an important part in controlling seasonal allergies. Sweets, dairy products, and cold foods all tend to increase mucus buildup, putting ice cream and yogurt at the top of the list of foods to avoid during allergy season. When excessive mucus accumulates in the system, allergens stimulate a much stronger allergic reaction. Soups, salads (in warm weather), vegetables, and boiled grains are all easy for the body to digest. When digestion is efficient, there is less of a tendency for mucus to build up.

Treatment plans for allergies vary greatly, and the possible results range from temporary relief to complete remission. Acupuncture frequently relieves allergy symptoms immediately. Manipulation of points around the nose, such as Yintang, Bitong, and Large Intestine 20, usually relieves the nasal congestion and sneezing as soon as the needles are inserted.

Recently, a similar but more sophisticated system of allergy-elimination acupuncture has been developed in which the acupuncture is performed while the person is exposed to the allergen. Developed by Dr. Devi Nambudripad, this technique is called Nambudripad's Allergy Elimination Technique (NAET). The patient undergoes allergy testing to identify the allergen. Then acupressure and acupuncture techniques are used to clear the allergen while the patient is exposed to it. This treatment reprograms the body to accept the allergen without producing an allergic reaction. The effects are long-term, and the allergy is virtually eliminated.

Arthritis

Arthritis is a degenerative inflammatory disease that attacks the joints in particular, causing symptoms of stiffness, swelling, pain, and loss of the normal range of motion. It is especially common in elderly people, although rheumatoid arthritis can occur in young people as well. In traditional Chinese patterns of disharmony, the various types of arthritis fall typically under the category of "painful obstruction syndrome." Acute painful obstruction can be due to wind, cold, dampness, or heat, although it is usually a combination of wind, dampness, and cold. In an acute attack of wind, cold, and dampness, symptoms include joint pain that gets worse with cold and is relieved with warmth, a feeling of

heaviness or numbness in the limbs, limited mobility of the affected area, and, possibly, a slow pulse. A more chronic arthritis condition is generally associated with an underlying deficiency of the vital substances involving the liver and kidneys, in view of their relationship to the tendons and bones.

The most common Western treatment for arthritis is nonsteroidal anti-inflammatory drugs (NSAIDS). Although these drugs can relieve pain and decrease inflammation, they do nothing to cure the disease. And their common side effect, gastric irritation, can lead to ulcers. In fact, a patient often bounces back and forth between a rheumatologist and gastroenterologist, first receiving treatment for the arthritis and then receiving treatment for the ulcer caused by the medication.

Traditional Chinese treatments also reduce pain and inflammation, but they focus on eliminating the cause of the arthritis and, thus, the disease itself. Arthritis responds very well to acupuncture. When combined with moxa, it can relieve pain and reduce inflammation immediately. Some acute cases require only a few treatments. Needles are typically placed into points surrounding the painful area, bringing circulation to the area and helping relieve the stagnation that causes pain and swelling. A more chronic, long-term arthritic condition can take months or even years to resolve. For this reason, it is essential to begin treating this disorder at the earliest stage possible.

Herbal therapy is especially important as part of the treatment of chronic cases. The treatment strategy varies, depending on whether the condition is due to heat or cold, or if there is a deficiency of any vital substances. Herbal remedies in chronic cases of cold and dampness need to nourish the underlying deficiency as well as expel the cold and dampness. The patent formula for this condition is **Du Huo Ji Sheng Wan**. The most effective formula is one custom-made for the patient's individual constitution and pattern of disharmony.

In any type of arthritis, it is important for the person to get regular exercise to warm the body and get the qi and blood flowing through the meridians. Since arthritis is a disorder involving stagnation, movement is an essential part of the healing process. If the pattern involves cold and dampness (the most common pattern), the diet should consist mostly of cooked foods with moderate amounts of warming anti-inflammatory spices such as cayenne and ginger. Although coffee is warming, it should be avoided due to its irritating nature.

Common Cold

The common cold has many forms in traditional Chinese medicine. The most common forms fall under the categories of wind cold and wind heat. As is the nature of exterior disorders involving wind, the pattern may change very quickly, necessitating a change in treatment strategy over the course of an illness. In all the forms a cold, as well as a cough or the flu, may take, prompt treatment brings the most effective results. The longer one waits to treat an infectious disease, the longer it takes to clear the pathogen.

Wind Cold: This pattern exhibits the following symptoms: fever, chills (these are worse than the fever), inability to get warm, nasal or sinus congestion with clear mucus, cough with clear mucus, stiff neck and shoulders, occipital headache (back of head), and a slower-than-normal pulse that is more easily felt at the surface. Diaphoretic (sweating) therapy is especially helpful in this condition, since it warms the body and pushes the pathogen out through the pores. In the very early stages of this pattern, an effective remedy is miso soup with the white part of spring onion (cong bai) and fresh ginger (sheng jiang). For more severe or advanced cases, there is a full range of therapies, depending on the combination of symptoms.

When the wind-cold symptoms include strong chills, inability to sweat, wheezing, and stiff neck, the classic and ancient remedy is Ephedra Decoction (Ma Huang Tang). The chief herb in this formula is Ephedra (ma huang), a powerful stimulant that opens the bronchial passages, warms the body, and stimulates sweating. Cinnamon twig (gui zhi) assists the Ephedra in warming the body and promoting a sweat, while apricot seeds (xing ren) help relieve the wheezing. Licorice (gan cao) acts as a harmonizing herb, modulating the harsh nature of the Ephedra, preventing too much sweating and toxicity. It also has anti-inflammatory and antitussive qualities, making it useful for sore throat and cough symptoms. Ephedra is never used by itself in Chinese herbal therapy; it is always part of a formula, often combined with licorice (as in Ephedra Decoction), which tones down its harsh nature. Since Ephedra can raise blood pressure, especially when used alone or with caffeine, it should not be used by people who have heart disease or hypertension.

For symptoms of wind cold with headache and nasal congestion as the chief symptoms, the classic formula is **Chuan Xiong Cha Tiao Wan**, typically taken with green tea (cha), which moves the action of the formula to the head area. Green tea has been found recently to have strong antioxidant properties, scavenging the free radicals involved in aging and disease.

Wind Heat: When the pernicious influence of wind combines with heat, the fever is worse than the chills, and the pulse is faster than normal. The primary symptom is a swollen and sore throat with headache and irritability. If there is a cough, it is usually dry or nonproductive, with occasional expectoration of yellow mucus. Numerous formulas treat the many variations of this condition, but the most famous by far is Yin Qiao San. This highly effective treatment for wind heat symptoms, appearing in such conditions as influenza and tonsillitis as well as the common cold, is also available from a number of different manufacturers as the patent formula **Yin Qiao Jie Du Pian**.

In addition to Yin Qiao, a number of effective remedies are discussed in the section on patent medicines (pages 191–248). For example, **Gan Mao Ling** is almost always useful in cases of wind heat. If the fever is high, **Zhong Gan Ling** is preferred. If the sore throat is especially severe, it is recommended to add **Chuan Xin Lian Antiphlogistic Tablets** to the treatment.

When treating cold or flu symptoms due to wind heat, the results are always more dramatic if the treatment begins at the earliest possible stage of the illness. It is important to get adequate rest, a vacation from sources of stress, and good nutrition in the form of soups and fresh juices. Sweets and stimulants (such as caffeinated beverages) cause a rapid progression in the severity of the illness since they tend to feed the pathogen. The same is true for tonifying herbs such as ginseng. People sometimes make the mistake of taking ginseng when they feel a cold coming on since they have heard that ginseng is good for the immune system. Using ginseng in this case is a serious error since ginseng will powerfully feed the pathogen causing the illness, making the person feel much worse. This is traditionally known as "trapping the burglar." If a person suspects a burglar is in the house, the worst step to take is to lock all the doors and windows, for the burglar will do more damage trying to get out. A powerful tonic herb, ginseng acts to "lock down" the exterior of the body while releasing energy in the interior. If a pathogen is already inside the body, ginseng and other stimulating tonics lock it in while simultaneously feeding it. The proper treatment plan is to open the pores and push out the pathogen. Herb formulas that "release the exterior and repel wind," such as Yin Qiao, are used in these cases.

On the other hand, if no pathogen is in the body, ginseng strengthens the wei qi, the body's wall against invaders, while it simultaneously improves the person's vitality and resistance to disease. This distinction between building long-term immunity and fighting off an acute illness is an important contribution of traditional Chinese medicine. While tonic herbs can be taken long-term, it is important to discontinue their use during a cold or flu. Then, after the pathogen has been expelled

from the body, tonic herbs can be taken again to build up strength and vitality over the long-term.

Acupuncture and moxibustion can provide some immediate relief from cold symptoms and help the body expel the pathogen much faster. Needles are typically inserted into points along the lung and large intestine meridians, which have demonstrated the ability to activate immune function. The most important acupuncture point in treating the common cold is Large Intestine 4 ("Adjoining Valleys"), which is located in the web between the thumb and index finger. This point is very effective for this condition, since it suppresses pain and relieves exterior conditions. Patients frequently experience quick relief when the point is needled or massaged. Typically, one or two acupuncture treatments and a week's course of herbal medicine are all that are required for colds. If the symptoms are recognized and treated early, it is possible to fight off a cold in a day or two with acupuncture treatment and herbs. (See also pages 171–174 for a discussion of the various types of coughs and their remedies.)

Constipation

If you notice a sudden change in your bathroom habits, have to strain to move your bowels, or feel uncomfortable even after you've attempted to have a bowel movement, you may be constipated, which happens when stools pass too slowly through your intestines. Constipation can have many causes, including not getting enough fluids, dietary fiber, or physical activity; not going to the bathroom when you feel the urge; use of certain drugs; and overuse of laxative. Constipation is also related to some serious health conditions such as depression, hyperthyroidism, and colon cancer.

A number of patterns of disharmony, both excess and deficiency, can cause constipation. The excess patterns are excess heat and qi stagnation. When exterior heat penetrates into the interior, it can affect the large intestine, with symptoms of high fever, thirst,

and sweating. The pulse is full and rapid, and the tongue is red with a yellow coat. In this case, herbs are selected that have a cooling, purgative effect such as rhubarb root (da huang). A simple but effective formula for this condition is Xiao Cheng Qi Tang ("Less Drastic Purgative Decoction"). The patent formula, **Peach Kernel Pills**, is an effective remedy for less severe cases of constipation due to excess heat.

Constipation due to stagnant qi typically gets worse when the person is under stress. In this case, herbs are given that relax stuck qi and restore intestinal function. A good combination of patent medicines to take for this pattern is **Xiao Yao Wan** and **Mu Xiang Shun Qi Wan**.

A deficiency of qi, blood, yin, or yang can also cause constipation. When qi is deficient, the person does not have the energy to move the bowels and often feels exhausted after trying. A person with this condition has a pale face and tongue and may break into a sweat while defecating. A good patent remedy for this condition is **Shen Qi Da Bu**

Wan, which contains qi tonics such as *Astragalus* (huang qi) and *Codonopsis* (dang shen). *Cannabis* seeds (huo ma ren) are a good addition, since they are a nourishing, lubricating laxative. They are now available in health food stores in the form of hemp seed oil. If yang is also deficient, the person feels cold and may have low back pain. In this case, the formula should also contain *Cistanches* (rou cong rong); the patient should eat walnuts (hu tao ren), a lubricating yang tonic.

If yin deficiency is the underlying cause, the person has small, hard, dry stools, thirst, night sweats, and a red tongue with little or no coating. The patent medicine **Rehmannia Teapills** with the addition of some hemp seed oil is appropriate in this pattern.

Acute constipation is relatively easy to resolve with one or two acupuncture treatments and herbal laxatives. The most important acupuncture point for this condition is Stomach 25 ("Heaven's Axis"), located on either side of the navel. Depending on the severity of the constipation, herbal laxatives ranging in strengths from mild lubricants to strong purgatives can usually bring relief within a day. Chronic constipation is typically due to a deficiency in one of the vital substances, making tonifying herbs the treatment of choice. The herbs and acupuncture points are selected according to which vital substance needs to be nourished. Fully correcting the imbalance can take anywhere from a few days to a few months, with a weekly acupuncture treatment acting to keep qi flowing through the intestines.

Cough

Traditional Chinese medicine is especially effective in the treatment of coughs because of its careful differentiation of the various types. For example, a cough due to heat produces sticky phlegm that is difficult to expectorate; it is treated with cooling, moistening herbs and acupuncture points that clear heat from the lungs. On the other hand, a cough due to cold is accompanied by chills and copious mucus; it is treated with warming, drying herbs and the application of moxibustion. Without this differentiation, it is easy to see how an unfocused treatment might be ineffective or even cause the cough to get worse. Descriptions of a few of the more commonly diagnosed types of coughs in Chinese medicine follow.

Hot Phlegm Cough: In this syndrome, the accumulated phlegm becomes thick and sticky due to heat. The cough can have a loud, barking sound. The phlegm is quite difficult to expectorate and the heat gives it a darker color, ranging from yellow to brown or dark green. This type of cough requires aggressive treatment as the green indicates that the trapped mucus has become infected. Mucus in the lungs is an ideal breeding ground for bacteria, so it is important to clear the mucus as quickly as possible with herbs that moisten the lungs to dislodge the mucus and stimulate expectoration. A highly effective formula for this condition is **Pinellia Expectorant Pills**. This patent medicine is available under several names, includ-ing Qing Qi Hua Tan Wan or Pinellia Root Teapills, but they are all the same formula. To maximize the effect, it is best to take it along with **Gan Mao Ling** or **Yin Qiao Jie Du Pian**.

As in all syndromes involving phlegm, diet is extremely important. It is best to avoid cold foods, dairy products, and sweets, as these all create mucus. Therapeutic foods include hot soups, cooked vegetables and whole grains, and small amounts of raw juices at room temperature to assist in moistening the lungs in order to promote expectoration.

Damp or Cold Phlegm Cough: This pattern is characterized by frequent coughing with expectoration of copious amounts of clear or sticky white phlegm that is typically more plentiful in the morning or after meals. There can also be nausea, a sensation of fullness in the chest or abdomen, poor appetite, fatigue, and a sensation of heaviness. The principle treatment in this syndrome is to clear the phlegm from the lungs and strengthen the digestion, since an underlying deficiency in spleen qi creates an inclination toward excessive mucus production. The classic formula for this condition is Er Chen Tang, or "Two Old Things Decoction," with the addition of herbs to repel the pathogen and warm the lungs. The patent version of Er Chen Tang is **Er Chen Wan**. If there are accompanying wind-cold symptoms of headache, stiff neck, and nasal congestion, the patent medicine **Chuan Xiong Cha Tiao Wan** can also be taken. Dietary therapy is similar to that for hot phlegm cough, except the avoidance of cold foods is especially important. A person with this condition should consume lots of hot liquids, especially ginger tea, get plenty of rest, and stay warm. Hot soup made mostly from vegetables is a tasty treatment as well.

Wind Dryness Cough: This type of cough is typically contracted after exposure to a dry environment. Different from a chronic dry cough caused by a deficiency of lung yin (often from smoking), in this case the dryness of the air allows the dryness external pernicious influence to attack the lungs. The symptoms are a dry cough and a sore throat with a ticklish sensation, dry lips and mouth, and, possibly, a headache. The treatment principle is to repel the dryness pernicious influence, moisten the lungs, and stop the cough. A classic formula for this condition is Sang Xing Tang (pronounced sahng shing tahng), translated as "Mulberry Leaf and Apricot Seed Decoction." This formula doesn't come in a patent medicine, but an effective replacement is **Chuan Bei Pi Pa Gao**. The diet should consist of soups and plenty of liquids. When the condition is gone, it would be wise to begin taking American ginseng (xi yang shen) on a daily basis for a few weeks. This will strengthen the qi and yin of the lungs and make a future attack less likely.

Most acute coughs respond to the above treatments within a week, unless the person fails to improve their diet and get some rest. In that case, the cough can linger for weeks, often leading to a series of colds due to weakened immunity. Acupuncture therapy is very helpful in treating coughs due to any cause. Needling a point on the Conception Vessel meridian (an extra meridian) just above the sternum can quickly calm a cough and assist breathing. Moxa therapy is used typically in the cold, damp type of cough, since there is a need for warmth in that pattern.

Diarrhea

The causes of diarrhea vary. In acute cases, a person can become dehydrated very quickly, so it is important to seek immediate medical attention if the condition persists. If an acute case of diarrhea occurs along with a common cold or stomach upset and it is accompanied by nausea, vomiting, and a lack of appetite, a reliable remedy is **Huo Xiang Zheng Qi Wan**.

If contaminated food or water is the cause, the diarrhea is often accompanied by a burning sensation and a strong smell. In these cases, a practitioner provides treatment to kill the pathogen (usually bacteria) with a formula such as **Huang Lian Su Pian** and restore normal digestive function with a formula such as **Mu Xiang Shun Qi Wan**. Most practitioners recommend a laboratory test to ensure the pathogens are eliminated.

In cases of chronic loose stools, the underlying pattern is usually spleen qi deficiency. Other symptoms might be fatigue, poor appetite, pale face and tongue, and gurgling sounds in the intestines. **Shen Ling Bai Zhu Pian** is an effective remedy in this pattern: The *Codonopsis* and *Atractylodes* herbs tonify the spleen, while its astringent herbs, such as lotus seeds, stop the diarrhea.

Acute diarrhea is fairly easy to treat with one or two acupuncture treatments and a few days of herbal therapy. Two points on the stomach meridian (25 and 37) are especially effective; relief comes soon after they are needled. If the diarrhea is chronic and due to qi or yang deficiency, moxibustion is very helpful when applied to these points. If the cause of discomfort is bacteria or parasites, herbal therapy as described above is the recommended treatment. The length of time needed to treat chronic cases varies; ultimately, the person's dietary habits are usually the decisive factor. Cases due to severe qi deficiency can take a few weeks to months to resolve.

In all types of diarrhea, it is important to drink sufficient liquids to avoid dehydration. Hot peppermint tea or vegetable broth are good choices. Plain white rice is the best solid food to soothe the stomach and firm up the stools until the condition passes.

Fatigue

Fatigue is a symptom of many different disorders, both psychological and physical. It is often difficult to discover its cause with modern Western diagnostic methods. Fortunately, diagnosing and treating this sort of generalized complaint is one of the strong points of Chinese medicine.

The first and most important step is to examine the person's lifestyle to eliminate any possible causes of fatigue, such as lack of sleep, poor diet, insuffi-cient exercise, or overworking. Without correcting these problems, it is difficult or impossible to restore the patient's energy level. Once the proper lifestyle adjustments are made, treatment, particularly moxibustion and herbal therapy, are much more likely to be effective.

The most common diagnoses in cases of chronic fatigue are deficiency of qi, blood, or yang, and many cases are a combination of these syndromes. In cases of qi deficiency, there may be no physical abnormality, but the body lacks sufficient energy to perform various functions. In addition to fatigue, the patient has a weak pulse, pale tongue, bright pale face, and, possibly, shortness of breath and poor appetite, depending on the organs involved. Most qi tonics boost energy by improving the function of the lungs, spleen, and kidneys. Some appropriate patent remedies to rectify qi deficiency are **Bu Zhong Yi Qi Wan**, **Nu Ke Ba Zhen Wan**, **Shen Qi Da Bu Wan**, **Extractum Astragali**, and **Ginseng Royal Jelly Vials**. Typically, these herbal remedies are taken for a few months, since chronic deficiency syndromes take longer to rectify. Acupuncture therapy is administered to bring energy to deficient organs, and moxibustion is applied to important systemic points to bring new energy into the body. Acupuncture points are selected that tonify the vital substances, since a deficiency of one or more of them is usually the underlying cause of fatigue. The most important tonifying points are Stomach 36, Spleen 6, Kidney 3, Du 4, and Ren 4. When these points are activated with acupuncture and moxa, the entire body becomes energized. (See "How to Moxa Stomach 36," page 143.) When combined with herbal therapy, a course of treatment typically takes place over a few weeks or months, depending on the severity of the problem.

In cases of blood deficiency, there is insufficient blood to nourish the organs and tissues of the body. In mild cases, the blood count may be within the normal range, while more severe cases are diagnosed as anemia, which can occur as a result of decreased bone marrow function, vitamin or iron deficiency, general malnutrition, blood loss from excessive menstrual flow, or an abnormal destruction of red blood cells.

In traditional Chinese medicine, anemia is associated with a deficiency of vital substances in the heart, liver, spleen, and kidneys. Herbal therapy and moxibustion are frequently successful in normalizing the blood count, no matter what the underlying pattern of disharmony is. Such therapy is closely monitored with regular blood tests, since anemia can have serious consequences if it persists. A typical course of treatment—a weekly acupuncture and moxa session and daily use of tonifying herbs—might take a few months. Two of the important acupuncture points for anemia are Spleen 10 ("Sea of Blood") and Stomach 36 ("Leg Three Miles"). Spleen 10 is chosen for its regulatory effect on the blood, while Stomach 36 improves the assimilation of nutrients from food, aiding in the production of new blood cells.

A deficiency of both spleen qi and heart blood produces dizziness, poor appetite, and fatigue, with a pale face and tongue. This pattern often appears in students after excessive studying. The standard formula for this pattern is **Kwei Be Wan**. In addition, longan (long yan rou) fruit can be eaten as is or boiled in a decoction. It is sold in dried form, but in tropical climates it can sometimes be found fresh. It nourishes the heart blood, making it a good supplement to herbal therapy.

If the underlying disharmony is liver and kidney yin deficiency, symptoms are fatigue, blurry vision, low back pain, sexual dysfunction, leg weakness, and night sweats. The treatment principle is to tonify liver and kidney yin with **Rehmannia Teapills**. Another tasty fruit, Lycium berries (gou qi zi), can be added as a supplement for this pattern. The berries replenish the yin of the liver and kidneys, nourish the blood, and improve eyesight. The best-quality fruit is brownish and soft and can be eaten as is, cooked into cereal, or boiled in a decoction.

When anemia is the result of spleen and kidney yang deficiency, fatigue, a pale face and tongue, lack of libido, cold limbs, and loose stools can occur. Moxibustion is especially helpful in this pattern. Also, the person should avoid cold foods. In this case, a good patent remedy is **Nu Ke Ba Zhen Wan**, which tonifies both qi and blood. In addition, a decoction made of 10 grams dried ginger and 10 grams cinnamon bark tonifies the yang qi.

In all types of anemia, another patent medicine, **Tang Kwei Gin**, a pleasant-tasting liquid supplement, further builds the blood. The diet should be especially nutritious, with generous amounts of dark greens and legumes at most meals. Refined foods such as pastas, breads, and pastries should be avoided, since they are filling but provide very little nutrition.

Headache

Headaches can occur in a variety of disease patterns in traditional Chinese medicine. Some headaches are associated with external pernicious influences, such as wind cold, wind heat, or wind damp. Others occur as a symptom of internal imbalances, such as liver fire, phlegm, blood stagnation, qi deficiency, or blood deficiency. It is especially important to have an accurate diagnosis when treating a headache, since the wrong treatment can actually make the condition worse.

When a headache is caused by an external pernicious influence, it can occur suddenly, often along with other symptoms of wind. When it is due to wind cold, the pain is typically in the back or the top of the head. Other symptoms could be an aversion to cold, tight and sore shoulders and neck, and nasal congestion. The classic formula for this pattern is **Chuan Xiong Cha Tiao Wan** taken along with green tea. When wind heat is the culprit, the headache can be quite severe. Other symptoms may be fever, sore throat, thirst, and a floating, rapid pulse. In this case, the appropriate formula is **Yin Qiao Jie Du Pian** or **Gan Mao Ling**. When the external pathogen is dampness, the pain is dull and the head feels heavy—as if it is wrapped in a wet

blanket. There can also be fever or chills, nasal congestion, foggy thinking, and fatigue. An effective patent remedy for this type of headache is **Huo Xiang Zheng Qi Wan**, which is also appropriate for headaches due to internal dampness. In all the above types of acute, externally contracted headaches, the pain may be due, in part, to pressure in the sinuses. If any nasal or sinus congestion accompanies the headache, it is a good idea to take **Bi Yan Pian** also.

A common internal cause of headache is liver yang rising up to the head, which may occur when a person experiences anger or frustration, or it can be a result of long-term deficiency of liver yin. Symptoms are dizziness, irritability, and nausea; the headache is a throbbing pain on the sides of the head or behind the eyes. The classic formula for this condition is Tian Ma Gou Teng Yin, which is also quite effective in relieving tight neck and shoulders that can accompany the headache. It contains two herbs specific for headaches due to liver imbalances. In the condition known as liver fire, a condition of extreme heat, the symptoms are the same as for liver yang headaches, with the addition of red face and eyes, more severe anger, and a red tongue with a yellow coat. The standard formula for this pattern is **Long Dan Xie Gan Wan**, which purges heat from the liver.

Symptoms of blood stagnation headaches are a sharp, fixed, stabbing pain in a specific location, a wiry, choppy pulse, and a purple tongue. Usually, previous traumatic injury caused the blood stagnation. Herbs are selected that move the blood and help to relieve pain, such as **Yan Hu Suo Zhi Tong Pian**.

A headache due to qi deficiency typically begins or gets worse after physical exertion, and it tends to feel better in the morning or after rest. A dull pain, it can be accompanied by fatigue and a poor appetite. The treatment principle in this case is to tonify qi. Some appropriate patent remedies are **Bu Zhong Yi Qi Wan** or **Shen Qi Da Bu Wan**.

If blood deficiency is the cause, the pain is dull but a little more severe than the pain of qi deficiency. A pale face and tongue, dizziness, blurry vision, and a small, thin pulse are typical symptoms. The pain begins or gets worse when the person is hungry or after the menstrual period. The classic formula, **Nu Ke Ba Zhen Wan**, tonifies qi and blood. Also, **Tang Kwei Gin** or **Shou Wu Chih** are effective blood tonics in a convenient, good-tasting liquid form.

In all types of headaches, acupuncture is a powerful tool, frequently relieving the pain within minutes. A point used for all types of headaches is Large Intestine 4 ("Adjoining Valleys"), since it relieves pain in general and is a specific point for conditions affecting the head. Other points are selected according to the location of the pain, such as the back of the head (Gallbladder 20), the temples (Taiyang), or the forehead (Stomach 8). Following the treatment, it is important to incorporate some lifestyle and dietary modifications to eliminate the underlying cause of the headaches. For example, when the cause is liver heat, spicy and greasy foods should be avoided, and stress reduction should be a high priority. If the underlying pattern is qi or blood deficiency, the diet should be modified to incorporate more whole grains and beans, nuts, dark greens, and fresh, organic vegetables. Animal products tonify qi and blood, but they should be eaten in smaller quantities than the other foods. The protein, fats, and other nutrients they contain make them useful in rebuilding the body in cases of deficiency, but these same qualities make them factors in heart disease and cancer when eaten in excess.

···

Indigestion

Overeating or combining foods that are difficult to digest leads to acute indigestion or a condition known in Chinese medicine as food stagnation. Symptoms include a lack of appetite and an aversion to food, a full, bloated feeling in the stomach, nausea, vomiting, bad breath, and acid belching. The treatment principle is to move qi in the stomach, thereby stimulating digestion and moving the contents of the stomach into

the intestines. In these cases, **Pill Curing** is especially effective.

Another possible cause of acute indigestion is eating while under stress: The liver becomes hyperactive and impairs the digestive function of the spleen. Treatment involves soothing the liver while simultaneously stimulating digestion, and an appropriate remedy is **Shu Gan Wan**.

Chronic weak digestion is commonly due to a deficiency of qi or yang in the spleen, the principal organ of digestion in traditional Chinese medicine. When the qi of the spleen is deficient, it is unable to perform its functions of digestion. In addition to the typical qi deficiency signs of fatigue and pale face and tongue, symptoms of chronic weak digestion include poor appetite, weight loss, fullness and sleepiness after eating, and loose stools. A useful remedy for this condition is **Six Gentlemen Teapills**, since it contains herbs that relieve indigestion along with herbs that strengthen spleen qi. If spleen yang is also deficient, all the same symptoms are present with the addition of cold hands and feet, a desire for warm food and drinks, abdominal pain and discomfort after eating cold foods, and diarrhea with undigested food in the stools. In this case, the above patent formula should be taken along with strong ginger tea. Ginger tea can be purchased in tea bags or made fresh by simmering slices of ginger root in water for a few minutes. The diet should consist primarily of soups and cooked foods but no cold or raw foods. Moxibustion to Stomach 36 and points on the abdomen also boosts the qi and yang of the spleen, gradually increasing the body's digestive strength.

Acute cases of indigestion are quite easy to treat, usually responding to one acupuncture treatment or a tube of **Pill Curing**. Chronic cases of indigestion due to an underlying spleen qi deficiency can take a few weeks to resolve. The classic point for all types of digestive weakness is Stomach 36, which responds equally well to moxa or acupuncture. If the person fails to change unhealthy dietary habits, the condition will be very difficult to treat.

水

Insomnia

Insomnia can occur as a result of excess conditions such as liver fire, heart fire, and food stagnation. It is also a symptom of deficiency, especially heart yin, blood, or qi deficiency. Although treatment for these conditions varies, most cases respond well to variations of **Emperor's Tea** since it has nourishing sedatives along with herbs that clear heat. A number of effective remedies for insomnia are available in the form of patent medicines, including **Emperor's Tea**, **An Mien Pien**, and **An Shen Bu Xin Wan**.

When insomnia occurs, lifestyle changes also help. As bedtime approaches, avoid stimulation by turning off most of the lights and staying away from televisions or computers. Going to bed either too full or too hungry can also disturb sleep patterns. Too many sweet foods or caffeinated beverages may also cause insomnia.

The possible treatment options for insomnia vary greatly, depending on the severity of the condition. Certain acupuncture points have strong sedating qualities, such as points on the wrist (Heart 7) and ear, both of which are named "Spirit Gate," as well as a point between the eyebrows (Yintang). When these points are needled, the brain releases natural opiates; the patient frequently falls asleep and wakes feeling relaxed and refreshed. Receiving an acupuncture treatment late in the day reduces stress and promotes restful sleep. Chronic insomnia requires herbal therapy that addresses the underlying condition, often consisting of herbs from the category of "substances that nourish the heart and calm the spirit."

Menstrual Pain

Painful menstruation can arise from a variety of causes, including emotional factors, cervical or uterine abnormalities, cysts or tumors, or endometriosis. In traditional Chinese medicine, most patterns are variations on deficiency or stagnation of qi and blood. When qi is more stagnant than blood, symptoms of premenstrual syndrome (PMS) and pain in the breasts, ribs, abdomen, and back can occur, along with a scanty menstrual flow with some clots. The treatment principle is to regulate qi, and the classic herbal formula for that is **Xiao Yao Wan**.

When blood is more stagnant than qi, symptoms include sharp abdominal pain that is relieved after the menstrual blood flow begins. The blood is darker than normal with dark clots. The classic formula for this pattern is Tao Hong Si Wu Tang ("Four Substance Decoction with Safflower and Peach Pit").

If the pattern is one of qi and blood deficiency, dull pain occurs after the menstrual flow is finished. The pain, which is relieved with pressure, may be accompanied by fatigue, pale face and tongue, dizziness, and a weak pulse. The standard formula to tonify qi and blood is Ba Zhen Tang ("Eight Precious Ingredients Decoction"). It is available as the patent remedy **Nu Ke Ba Zhen Wan**. In all cases of menstrual pain, **Yan Hu Suo Zhi Tong Pian** can be used along with the other herbs to help relieve the pain.

Acute menstrual pain can sometimes be relieved with just a single acupuncture treatment, depending on the severity of the underlying pattern of disharmony. If there is pain due to stagnation from cold, moxibustion also provides immediate relief. In chronic cases, it usually takes up to three months or more for the cycle to return to normal.

Premenstrual Syndrome

Premenstrual syndrome (PMS) is a common condition that occurs in the seven to ten days before menstruation and disappears shortly after bleeding begins. Caused by fluctuations in the hormonal balance of estrogen and progesterone, its symptoms include nervousness, irritability, emotional ups and downs, depression, water retention, and sore breasts.

From the point of view of Chinese patterns of disharmony, all of these symptoms can be traced to a stagnation of liver qi. Since the liver stores the blood and regulates the smooth flow of qi, it is almost always the organ involved in menstrual problems. When liver qi flows smoothly, the menstrual cycle is also smooth. The classic herbal formula for liver qi stagnation is **Xiao Yao Wan**. It is taken daily until bleeding begins, discontinued until menstruation is complete, and then taken daily again. This schedule is followed for three or four months; then a break is taken for a month. If symptoms persist, another three-month course of treatment can be undertaken. This is one of the most commonly prescribed of all the Chinese traditional formulas, and many women have experienced great relief from its use. It is also appropriate for men with symptoms of liver qi stagnation such as nervousness, irritability, and depression.

Acupuncture and moxibustion therapy are also highly effective in treating PMS symptoms. Often, a patient experiences complete relief while still in the practitioner's office. A powerful point known as "Great Pouring" (Liver 3) is often needled with powerful effects. This point can also be massaged by a person experiencing PMS symptoms or simply the stress of everyday life. Although acupuncture relieves acute symptoms quickly, chronic cases usually require two or three months of weekly acupuncture and daily herbal therapy before the condition is resolved.

Dietary therapy involves avoiding all sweets, strong spices such as hot peppers, and stimulants, especially coffee, which heats the liver and can actually cause this condition. Avoiding stress at this time also helps balance the energy of the liver.

Prostatitis

Prostatitis is an inflammation of the prostate gland often due to an acute bacterial infection. A urinary tract infection often accompanies prostatitis. Prostatitis symptoms include difficulty urinating, frequent urge to urinate, and pain in the prostate area. In acute cases of prostatitis, either acupuncture or herbs can provide immediate relief, while chronic cases take longer to resolve, depending on the severity of

the condition. Conventional Western treatment is antibiotic therapy, bed rest, and consumption of adequate fluids. In Chinese medicine, treatment of this condition, which corresponds to the pattern of lower burner damp heat, is the same as in acute urinary tract infections: Ba Zheng San. An herb that is especially effective in acute prostatitis is Vaccaria seed (wang bu liu xing). It is the chief ingredient in the patent medicine **Prostate Gland Pills**, an effective remedy for this condition.

Chronic prostatitis is often the result of deficiency of yin, yang, or qi in the kidneys. Treatment is **Rehmannia Six Teapills**, to which a practitioner often adds herbs specific to the patient's constitution and complaint. If there is a deficiency of yang, warm herbs such as aconite root (fu zi) and cinnamon bark (rou gui) are added.

Sciatica

In sciatica, pain travels from the buttocks down the back of the leg, following the course of the sciatic nerve.

Sciatica is usually caused by a lower back disk injury, usually a slipped disk pressing on the nerve; it's also possible that the nerve compression is in the pelvis or buttocks. Acupuncture is exceptionally effective for this condition: Many people experience immediate relief. Points are selected along the course of the sciatic nerve. The most important points are located on the gallbladder meridian and urinary bladder meridians. If sciatic pain is due to a severe injury to a spinal disk, treatment can take months and sometimes only brings partial relief. Moxibustion is also very helpful, as long as there is no underlying heat condition. The patent medicine **Sciatica Pills** is also quite effective in relieving the pain and inflammation. If there is accompanying low back pain, **Du Huo Ji Sheng Wan** can also be taken.

Sinusitis

This uncomfortable condition can be caused by a bacterial, fungal, or viral infection, or it can arise from an allergic reaction. Depending on the sinus cavities involved, pain occurs in the forehead, between the eyes, or in the mouth area. Typically, there is a yellow or green discharge from the nose, often dripping into the throat. In addition to the pain, the head feels heavy. The condition can become chronic, especially when a person has repeated colds. Unless a person gets sufficient rest, avoids mucus-forming foods, and recovers fully, the sinuses will not drain completely. It is important to treat this condition as early and aggressively as possible to prevent a serious infection that requires antibiotic treatment. A vicious cycle of repeated infections and antibiotic use can develop, further weakening the immune system and making the person more prone to future infections.

Traditional diagnostic patterns for sinusitis are wind cold, wind heat, lung heat, or liver and gallbladder fire that has ascended to the head. While each pattern has a different treatment, herbs and acupuncture points are used in all the patterns.

Acute conditions respond to acupuncture and herbal therapy within a few days. Needling points alongside the nose, such as Large Intestine 20 and the extra points Bitong or Yintang, is exceptionally effective at clearing the nasal passages and sinuses. These points are a little painful for about a second or two, but the discomfort is usually rewarded with an immediate clearing of the nasal passages and sinuses. Other points are selected according to the specific pattern of disharmony underlying the sinus problem.

A good base herbal formula for the practitioner to work from is Xanthium Powder (cang er san), which comprises *Xanthium* fruit (cang er zi), magnolia flower (xin yi hua), *Angelica dahurica* root (bai zhi), and field mint or peppermint (bo he). Since this formula is on the warm side, some cooling herbs such as honeysuckle flowers (jin yin hua) and *Scutellaria* root (huang qin) are added when signs of heat (fever or yellow mucus) are present. An appropriate patent medicine is **Bi Yan Pian** for the nasal and sinus congestion, along with a heat-clearing formula such as **Chuan Xin Lian Antiphlogistic Pills**.

Diet is especially important in any disharmony involving mucus, since many foods tend to increase it. The patient should avoid cold, greasy, and excessively spicy foods. Sweets make the condition worse, sometimes with immediate feedback from the sinuses in the form of more congestion and pain. Once an acute attack has been cleared, *Codonopsis* root (dang shen) or *Astragalus* root (huang qi), herbs that tonify the spleen, should be taken. They can be found in patents such as **Shen Qi Da Bu Wan**. When spleen qi is strong, less mucus is produced, and the immune system is better able to fight off the colds that lead to sinusitis.

Sore Throat

Sore throat can be acute or chronic. Acute cases are typically due to wind heat, with accompanying symptoms of fever, possibly a cough with yellow phlegm, and a floating, rapid pulse. The classic formula for this diagnosis is **Yin**

Qiao Jie Du Pian. The sooner it is taken once symptoms arise, the more quickly and effectively it clears the condition. If the sore throat is especially severe, add **Chuan Xin Lian Antiphlogistic Pills**. If the sore throat continues to get worse, seek medical attention immediately to determine if the condition is a strep infection.

Acute sore throats usually subside after a day or two of herbal therapy and acupuncture. The most commonly used points are Large Intestine 4 and Large Intestine 11 ("Crooked Pool"), located on the hand and arm. If the pain is especially severe, a point near the base of the thumb on the palm side (Lung 10) is very effective. Since this point can be painful to needle, it is usually reserved for more severe throat pain. In these cases, the patient is willing to tolerate a little extra discomfort from the needles in order to get relief from the throat pain.

A chronic sore throat can have yin deficiency as the underlying cause, since the lack of cooling yin can lead to chronic inflammation. Other symptoms of yin deficiency are a thin, rapid pulse, red tongue with little or no coating, dry mouth, night sweats, and irritability or insomnia. The treatment principle is to tonify yin and clear the heat with standard formulas such as **Rehmannia Teapills**. It might be necessary to take the formula for a few months for it to have a long-term effect.

Stress

Modern, industrialized societies run at such a fast pace, constant stress and anxiety are often considered by many people to be normal aspects of life. Many people won't even realize they're under stress until they are diagnosed with a stress-related condition such as high blood pressure or they have a stroke or heart attack. Of course, the best way to deal with stress is to eliminate as many possible sources of it as possible. Stress-reduction techniques such as qi gong, meditation, yoga, exercise, or spiritual practices can greatly lessen the effects of stress on both the mind and body.

The effects of acupuncture in reducing stress are truly remarkable. Patients always seem to be more relaxed and emotionally calm after a treatment. Certain points have especially calming effects, making them effective in treating insomnia, addictions, and anxiety disorders. In some cases, a practitioner may tape a small seedlike bead to a point on the ears known as "Spirit Gate." The person can then stimulate this point by pressing on the bead, helping maintain the calming effects of the acupuncture treatment.

Some patent remedies used for their calming effects are **Emperor's Tea** or **An Mien Pien**. Stronger extracts to reduce anxiety or induce sleep can also be obtained through practitioners. Zizyphus Seed Stress/Sleep Formula, a concentrated liquid extract, is very fast-acting and effective for stress or insomnia, depending on the dosage.

In addition, some herbs, known as adaptogens, help the body withstand the effects of stress. These include tonifying herbs such as ginseng, *Astragalus*, *Codonopsis*, and reishi mushroom.

Researched extensively in Russia and China, the effectiveness of these herbs as adaptogens is well documented. Some patents that contain adaptogens are **Ginseng Royal Jelly Vials**, **Extractum Astragali**, and **Kwei Be Wan**. A highly concentrated Siberian ginseng solid extract from Gaia herbs is also available in health food stores. It is very tasty in its honey base, and the feelings of well-being and higher energy levels can be felt soon after ingesting the extract.

Urinary Tract Infection

Although commonly called a bladder infection, a urinary tract infection (UTI) may be caused by bacteria in any part of the urinary tract, including the kidneys, ureters (the tubes that carry urine to the bladder from the kidneys), urethra (the tube that empties the bladder during urination), or bladder (the sac that "holds" urine before it is released through the urethra). The bacteria that cause UTIs most often enter the urethra and travel up through the urinary tract. Although men can experience infections of the urinary tract, women are much more likely to get them, for a number of reasons. First, because a woman's urethra is shorter than a man's, bacteria can more easily reach the bladder. Second, expectant mothers may be at higher risk for infections of the kidneys because a fetus can put pressure on the ureters. Finally, the act of sexual intercourse can push bacteria into the urethra. Wearing a diaphragm can put pressure on the urethra and make it harder for a woman to completely empty her bladder, causing bacteria to collect and flourish in the uneliminated urine.

The symptoms of UTI are the same for men and women: Frequent, painful urination and some difficulty when urinating (you feel the urge to go, but are able to void only a small amount). UTIs can be acute or chronic. A number of factors increase a person's risk of UTI, such as a new sexual partner, a diet high in carbohydrates and low in protein, and not drinking enough water.

The underlying pattern of chronic UTIs in traditional Chinese medicine is usually kidney yin deficiency. Other symptoms include a red tongue with very little coating, and, possibly, irritability and night sweats. With the cooling aspect of the kidneys depleted, the heat generated by yin deficiency can lead to a chronic inflammation. Western medicine treats UTIs with antibiotics, but unless the underlying yin deficiency is rectified, as soon as a person gets rid of one infection with antibiotics, another one sets in. This cycle can be repeated over and over, causing other problems from the side effects of the drugs. In Chinese medicine, the standard treatment for chronic UTI is to tonify yin and clear heat with a formula such as **Zhi Bai Di Huang Wan**.

The most common pattern associated with an acute UTI is damp heat in the urinary bladder. Symptoms are fever, possibly chills, burning urine, pain in the back or lower abdomen, an urgent need to urinate frequently, a red tongue with a thick yellow coat in the back, and a full, slippery pulse. An infection

Chinese Healing Secrets

at this stage is best treated by a practitioner, since the infection can easily become more serious and spread through the kidneys. A patent medicine that sometimes works at this stage is **Long Dan Xie Gan Wan**. A strong decoction using the traditional formula known as Ba Zheng San ("Eight Ingredient Powder to Correct Urinary Disturbances") is often recommended.

Acute cases often respond very quickly to acupuncture and herbs, sometimes in just a few days or even sooner. The most effective acupuncture point is Ren 3 ("Middle Summit"), located directly over the urinary bladder. Another important point is Spleen 9 ("Yin Tomb Spring"), located below the knee along the inside of the tibia bone. This point is often sensitive to pressure if there is a UTI, and it is very useful for all types of imbalances of the urinary tract. Its traditional functions are to transform damp stagnation and benefit the lower burner.

During therapy for UTIs, it is important to avoid sweets completely. Eat a protein source at every meal to make the urine more acidic and less hospitable to bacteria. Wear cotton underwear to ensure that air circulates and prevents a damp environment. Abstaining from sexual activity is advised, but if not feasible, both partners should shower before having intercourse to avoid further infiltration of bacteria into the urinary tract.

CHAPTER 11:
Chinese Herbal Patent Medicines

In China, herbal medicine is an integral part of mainstream society. Just as many Americans turn to over-the-counter medications for minor ailments, people in China have hundreds of herbal formulas available for a wide range of health problems. To fully explain the use of individual herbs and the art of herbal formulation is beyond the scope of this book. For this reason, this section describes patent medicines, which are already formulated for specific ailments and ready to take. This section introduces some of the best patent medicines for your home first-aid kit.

Patent medicines are an inexpensive and convenient way to administer Chinese medicinal herbs. Most of the patents come in the form of easy-to-swallow, tiny round pills (wan) or tablets (pian), plasters (gao), liquid extracts (zhi), or wine (jiu). Some of these highly effective remedies have been made by the same family for generations; many are based on traditional formulas that have been in use for more than two thousand years.

In most cases, people in the United States are introduced to patent remedies or other herbal formulas when they receive them from a traditional Chinese medicine practitioner as part of a course of treatment. Currently, patent medicines are rarely available in health food stores in the United States except in large cities and "alternative communities" such as Santa Cruz, California; Boulder, Colorado; or Santa Fe, New Mexico. However, as more people become interested in Chinese herbalism, the patents will begin to show up in more places, and they are available from mail-order sources. The most reliable source of patent formulas at this time is Mayway (see Resources, page 250). It imports the Plum Flower line of remedies, which is manufactured without any artificial colors, additives, or contaminants. It also imports the high-quality patents made at the Tianjin and Lanzhou Foci factories. These facilities manufacture formulas according to Good Manufacturing Procedures (GMP), which ensure high standards of cleanliness and quality control. In compliance with this industry standard, raw herbs are tested before production in order to ensure that they have their essential costituents and their essential qualities. In addition, the herbs are screened for mold, heavy metals, bacteria, and yeast. Since there are a number of counterfeit products

Some of the patent medicines that are available have been made by the same family for generations, and many of them are based on traditional formulas that have been in use in China for more than two thousand years.

on the market containing inferior ingredients and of questionable quality, Mayway makes sure it receives only the products from factories that adhere to GMP. It also works with organic farms in China and always attempts to find the highest quality herbs available. Mayway, therefore, is the recommended source for purchasing patents.

As is true for all types of home health care, these remedies are used to supplement professional medical care or as first-aid treatments. In no way should they substitute for professional medical treatment. Consult a skilled herbal practitioner before using these formulas. Remember that although herbal patents are natural, they have strong actions on the body and must be used according to specific guidelines and for specific symptoms. In the absence of a professional diagnosis or if there is any doubt about the condition, it is better to take no herbs at all rather than take the wrong ones. In most cases, the wrong patent formula will not have serious side effects, but the body can behave in unexpected ways.

Follow these general guidelines for use:

- Do not exceed the recommended dose.
- Do not use during pregnancy.
- Keep out of reach of children.

Herbs can have a stronger effect on children, the elderly, or those who are debilitated, so dosages should be decreased for use by them. When calculating dosages for children, assume an adult weighs 150 pounds. Decrease proportionally to the child's weight. For example, if an adult dose is 12 pills, the dosage for a 50-pound child should be one-third that, or 4 pills. Children younger than 1 year should not be given herbal medicine without the advice of a practitioner experienced in pediatrics.

Take the patents with water (warm water aids assimilation). Bear in mind that patents are made with herbs, which are, in fact, a type of food; so, the amount taken at one time will be larger than what you may be used to. For example, a dose of a prescription or over-the-counter drug is usually 1 to 2 pills whereas in Chinese medicine a dose is more likely to be 8 to 12 pills.

A person with a sensitivity to one or more ingredients in a patent may develop an allergic reaction. Symptoms include skin rash, itching, difficulty breathing, diarrhea, constipation, or stomachache. If any of these symptoms occurs, discontinue use immediately. If symptoms persist, seek medical care.

The patent medicines described in the following section are grouped according to their actions. For each patent, the most commonly used name appears first. A guide to its pronunciation follows its Chinese name (within parentheses), and the English translation of the Chinese name appears last (within quotation marks). When a patent is made by more than one factory, the most reputable manufacturer is listed. When purchasing patent medicines yourself, read labels carefully to be sure you're getting high quality herbs: Manufacturers of lesser quality herbs often copy the packaging of the reputable factories, so look for the full name of the manufacturer on the label.

Chinese Healing Secrets

Bi Yan Pian
(bee yahn pyen);
"Nose Inflammation Pills"

Indications: Acute or chronic nasal congestion, allergies, runny nose due to common cold

Functions: Dispels wind cold or wind heat, clears the nasal passages

Description: Bi Yan Pian is one of the more popular over-the-counter medicines. It is highly effective for nasal or sinus congestion as in the common cold, allergies, rhinitis, and sinusitis. The major herbal decongestants in this formula are magnolia flower (xin yi hua), *Angelica dahurica* (bai zhi), and *Xanthium* (cang er zi). These three herbs are effective individually, but their synergistic effect upon the nasal passages and sinuses is nothing short of remarkable. After prescribing this remedy dozens of times over the years, the only side effect one experienced practitioner has seen is some dryness in the mouth and throat. This occurred in only two cases, and it was alleviated by decreasing the dose. This example points to the need for assessing each case and prescribing an herbal remedy based on the individual's constitution. The individuals who experienced excessive dryness both had an underlying yin deficiency, which means that their body's ability to maintain a moist environment was impaired. Herbs that have a drying nature, as in this formula, tend to push that imbalance even further.

Bi Yan Pian can be used for sinus infections; it contains heat-clearing herbs such as *Phellodendron* (huang bai), forsythia (lian qiao), *Anemarrhena* (zhi mu), and wild chrysanthemum (ye ju hua). When treating an infection, it is best to be as aggressive as possible, since it can quickly progress to a more serious condition. For this reason, this patent formula is often combined with one that focuses more on clearing infections such as Chuan Xin Lian Antiphlogistic pills. In addition, when treating any infection with herbs, it is essential to begin taking the herbs as early as possible, take them regularly until the infection is gone, and then continue them for a day or two after the symptoms are gone. This last step is important because if treatment is discontinued early, it is possible to kill off enough bacteria to alleviate symptoms while still leaving enough behind to multiply again. Once an infection has been partially cleared with herbs and allowed to come back, it is much more difficult to clear it with the same herbs in a second round of treatment.

Until recently, the disadvantage of using Bi Yan Pian has been the presence of artificial dyes in the tablet coating. Some of the batches also contained traces of Western over-the-counter pharmaceuticals. This disturbing issue has been resolved in the Plum Flower line of patent medicines. This product line is manufactured without any artificial colors, Western drugs, or adulterants. Eventually, most of the popular remedies will be available through Plum Flower.

Manufacturer: Plum Flower

Dosage: 3 to 4 pills, three times a day. Do not exceed the recommended dosage because this formula contains *Xanthium*, which is slightly toxic.

Chuan Bei Pi Pa Gao
(*chwahn bay pee pah gow*);
"Fritillaria Loquat Syrup"

Indications: Cough due to lung heat or dryness, with phlegm that is difficult to expectorate; a dry cough with no or little phlegm

Functions: Clears lung heat, moistens the lungs, stops coughing

Description: This soothing syrup is appropriate in cases of lung dryness that is due to wind heat, common colds, or smoking. Its chief ingredients are Fritillaria (bei mu) and loquat leaf (pi pa ye). Loquat leaf is especially useful for a heat-type cough, which is a cough with sticky phlegm that is difficult to expectorate. Loquat leaf comes from the same tree that produces the small delicious loquat fruits (Eriobotrya japonica). Fritillaria, the other chief ingredient, is an expectorant that is moistening to the lungs, an important action when a cough is nonproductive.

Manufacturer: Nin Jom Manufactory

Dosage: 1 tablespoon, three times a day

Chuan Xin Lian Antiphlogistic Tablets (chwahn shin lyahn); "Andrographis Anti-inflammatory Tablets"

Indications: Inflammation due to excess heat, swollen glands, severe sore throat, viral infections, bacterial infections

Functions: Clears heat, clears toxins, cools the blood, reduces inflammation

Description: This powerful antibacterial and antiviral formula contains just three herbs: Andrographis leaf, Isatis root, and Taraxacum root (dandelion). The combination of these ingredients produces a pronounced cooling effect on toxic heat throughout the body. Some of the bacterial infections this patent medicine treats are acute sore throat, swollen glands, lung abscess, pneumonia, urinary tract infections, and dysentery. It can also be used for viral infections such as influenza and hepatitis.

The chief ingredient, Andrographis paniculata (chuan xin lian), has been shown to inhibit the Staphylococcus, Streptococcus, and Shigella organisms that can cause various infections. It is extremely bitter—its name in Chinese translates to "pierce the heart lotus," meaning it is so bitter, its flavor "pierces the heart." One herbalist recalls that while working in a Chinese herbal pharmacy some years ago, he noticed an extremely bitter taste in his mouth. When he turned around, he saw that a teacher had opened the drawer containing the *Andrographis*, 20 feet from where he was standing! Because of its bitterness, *Andrographis* is usually taken in pill form.

The second ingredient, *Isatis tinctoria* (ban lang gen), also has antiviral and antibacterial actions. Its broad antimicrobial effect has been shown to inhibit the bacteria that cause dysentery, salmonella, strep infection, and typhoid. *Isatis* has strong antiviral action against hepatitis and encephalitis. This is highly significant, since Western medicine has virtually no weapons against viral infections.

The third ingredient is the much-maligned dandelion (pu gong ying), a major medicine in both Western and Chinese herbalism. Traditionally used for breast abscesses,

jaundice, and urinary tract infections, dandelion has impressive antibacterial effects against the pathogens that cause strep throat, pneumonia, dysentery, meningitis, diphtheria, and tuberculosis—all from a plant that is relentlessly sprayed with herbicides by the unsuspecting suburban homeowner!

Manufacturer: United Pharmaceutical Manufactory

Dosage: 3 to 6 pills, three times a day

Chuan Xiong Cha Tiao Wan (*chwahn shuhng chah tyow wahn*); "Ligusticum and Green Tea Pills"

Indications: Headache and nasal congestion due to wind cold

Functions: Relieves headache and expels wind cold

Description: This remedy is specifically indicated for a headache along with wind cold symptoms of the common cold, such as stiff neck and shoulders, nasal congestion, a desire for warmth, and a slower than normal pulse. It is meant to be taken along with green tea, which helps maximize the healing action of the other herbs. Recent research has shown that green tea also has strong antioxidant properties, meaning it helps break down free radicals, substances involved in the aging and disease processes.

The chief herb in the formula is Ligusticum wallichii (chuan xiong), a highly aromatic plant with strong circulatory properties. A strong analgesic (pain reliever), it relieves the headaches that occur with a cold, and it is used in many herbal formulas to direct the formula's action to the head. Another ingredient is Notopterygium root, a fragrant herb that releases tension in the muscles of the shoulders and neck. Since the trapezius muscles extend from the upper back to the neck and head, tightness in that muscle group can lead to an occipital headache (the back of the head at the base of the skull). The inclusion of Angelica dahurica root (bai zhi) has the dual function of clearing sinus and nasal congestion and relieving the pain of frontal headaches (pain in the forehead). Wild ginger (xi xin) is another analgesic herb in the formula that acts as a decongestant. Its North American relative grows in the coastal redwood forests of California; when chewed, its gingery flavor quickly numbs the tongue, demonstrating its ability to act as a local anesthetic.

Chuan Xiong Cha Tiao Wan is also useful in dizziness and loss of balance due to labyrinthitis, an inflammation of the inner ear, a very uncomfortable condition that can follow a viral or bacterial infection. This patent's ability to increase circulation to the head helps facilitate healing in this ailment, for which there is no conventional treatment.

Since it is very warming, this remedy should not be used for headaches due to wind heat with symptoms such as sore throat, fever, and a faster than normal pulse or headaches due to liver heat rising to the head with its symptoms of rapid pulse, red face, and anger. It should also not be used when the headache is caused by a deficiency condition such as deficient qi, deficient blood, or deficient yin.

Manufacturer: Lanzhou Foci

Dosage: 8 pills, three times a day

Er Chen Wan
(*uhr chen wahn*);
"Two Old-Medicine Pills"

Indications: Excessive phlegm in the lungs and stomach with nausea, cough with abundant clear mucus

Functions: Regulates qi, reduces phlegm and dampness, harmonizes the stomach

Description: The two "old medicines" referred to in the name are aged citrus peel (chen pi) and *Pinellia* tuber (ban xia). The quality of these herbs is considered to improve with age. In fact, *Pinellia* is considered toxic until it is aged and treated with ginger. Citrus peel, the other chief ingredient, is a delightful medicinal with a sweet fragrance that is especially pronounced in the high-quality aged tangerine peels. Before you throw away the peel on a citrus fruit, you should know that citrus peel acts as an expectorant; increases secretion of gastric juices, which aids digestion; and has antibacterial effects.

This patent formula is indicated for a damp phlegm cough, which is associated with expectoration of copious amounts of clear or light-colored phlegm. In addition to their drying, expectorant activity, the two chief herbs in the formula alleviate the vomiting and nausea that sometimes accompany this condition. If the cough is due to the common cold, take this patent along with a formula such as Gan Mao Ling that helps eliminate the pathogen that caused the cold.

Manufacturer: Lanzhou Foci

Dosage: 8 pills, three times a day

Gan Mao Ling
(gahn mao ling);
"Cold Formula"

Indications: Cold or flu due to either wind heat or wind cold with fever, mild chills, sore throat, and stiff neck

Functions: Expels wind, clears heat, expels viruses

Description: Its extraordinary effectiveness makes Gan Mao Ling an extremely popular patent. You can use it to prevent a cold when you've been exposed to someone with a cold or to clear a cold or flu when it has already taken hold. In many cases, a few doses of Gan Mao Ling at the first sign of cold symptoms completely alleviates all symptoms, but it is also frequently all that is needed to relieve full-blown cold symptoms. It is an excellent base formula since it is effective in both cold and heat illnesses. If symptoms include nasal and sinus congestion, the formula can be taken with Bi Yan Pian. If a sore throat occurs along with the cold, it can be taken with Chuan Xin Lian Antiphlogistic Pills. If there is accompanying nausea or diarrhea, Curing Pills or Lophanthus Antifebrile (Huo Xiang Zheng Qi Wan) can be added.

This is another patent remedy that has been adulterated in the past with artificial coloring and Western pharmaceuticals. Once again, Plum Flower brand makes this important medicine available in a pure, unadulterated form. It is one of the essential patents for a first-aid kit.

Manufacturer: Plum Flower

Dosage: 3 to 6 pills, three times a day; to prevent a cold after exposure to someone with cold symptoms, take 2 tablets, three times a day for three days.

Lo Han Kuo Infusion,
Luo Han Guo Chong Ji
(law hahn gwaw chung jee);
"Momordica Fruit Instant Tea"

Indications: Cough due to lung heat or lung dryness, perhaps accompanied by sticky or bloody phlegm

Functions: Clears lung heat, moistens the lungs, stops cough

Description: Luo Han Guo ("smiling Buddha fruit") is the active ingredient in this instant tea. This exotic fruit is round with a brittle, egglike shell, which, when cracked open, reveals a clump of sweet seeds. The overall action of the fruit is nourishing and moistening, making it ideal for dryness in the lungs with an unproductive cough. This patent comes in the form of cubes that dissolve in water to make a pleasant-tasting tea. The formula's sweet taste makes it especially popular with children.

Manufacturer: Luo Han Guo Products Manufactory

Dosage: one cube dissolved in one cup of boiling water, two to three times a day

Ma Hsing Chih Ke Pien (*mah shing jih keh pyen*); "Ephedra Apricot Stop Cough Tablets"

Indications: Cough, bronchitis, or asthma due to heat

Functions: Clears lung heat, relieves asthma, stops cough

Description: Although this formula is used mostly to treat bronchitis with yellow phlegm due to heat, it is also quite effective in mild cases of asthma. The continual increase in the number of Americans with asthma could be due to such causes as air pollution, chemical exposure, or increased stress. Many people with asthma rely on chemical inhalers throughout the day, and some are forced to seek treatment in hospital emergency rooms on a regular basis for acute asthma attacks. Herbal medicine is quite effective in treating asthma. The results of herbal therapy range from a complete remission of the disease to a much less frequent use of inhalers.

The word ma in this formula's name refers to ma huang, or *Ephedra sinica*. This powerful herb contains ephedrine, a strong stimulant that dilates (widens) the bronchial tubes. During an asthma attack, the bronchial tubes narrow, causing a severe restriction in air flow. Inhalers open the passages to enable the person to breathe; *Ephedra* also handles the job well. When used properly, *Ephedra* is quite safe. Unfortunately, some products on the market exploit *Ephedra* as a stimulant for weight loss or recreational use, and deaths have occurred from overdoses of products that mix high levels of ephedrine and caffeine. This is a gross misuse of an important medicine. The U.S. Food and Drug Administration (FDA) is looking into the sale of these products; some states have already banned products containing high levels of ephedrine. Reputable, qualified practitioners in the United States hope the irresponsible actions of some manufacturers won't cause the removal of this valuable drug from the marketplace.

Ma Hsing Chih Ke Pien can also be used for cough due to heat, with sore throat, dry loud cough, or swollen glands. When used for chronic asthma, it is best to combine it with Ping Chuan Pills, which also contain herbs that tone and strengthen the lungs. In a clinical trial in China, the bulk version of this formula was given to 40 children with asthma. All of them experienced temporary relief; out of the 19 who had chronic asthma, only two children experienced relapses up to six months later.

Warning: *Ephedra* can raise blood pressure and should not be taken by people with high blood pressure, heart disease, a history of stroke, or a sensitivity to caffeine. Some people experience insomnia if they take the remedy too close to bedtime. Do not exceed recommended dosages. Asthma is a life-threatening condition for many people. While herbal medicine can greatly help in its treatment, be sure to keep an inhaler available for emergencies, even if it seems that you no longer need it.

Manufacturer: Siping Pharmaceutical Works

Dosage: 4 pills, two to three times a day

Minor Bupleurum,
Xiao Chai Hu Tang Wan
(show cheye hoo tahng wahn);
"Minor Bupleurum Pills"

Indications: Frequent colds and ear infections, colds with alternating fever and chills, malaria

Functions: Harmonizes the interior and exterior of the body, regulates the liver

Description: This patent fits easily in a number of formula categories. In Japan, where herbal formulas from China have become exceptionally popular over the past 20 years, Minor Bupleurum is the formula most frequently prescribed by medical doctors. It is used to stimulate the immune system, to treat hepatitis, and to protect against the side effects of radiation therapy. It has antiallergy activities and is also used to treat prolonged flu and colds as well as chronic digestion problems.

Take the case of a man who had just returned from traveling in Indonesia. He was experiencing a headache and extreme weakness, with chills, fever, and sweats. From a Western diagnostic perspective, he was exhibiting all the classic signs of malaria; from the traditional Chinese point of view, he was experiencing a shao yang condition, a clear indicator for Minor Bupleurum. Since this was a serious illness, he was given the formula in the form of a decoction, three times a day. After three days, his symptoms completely disappeared. About three months later, the symptoms appeared again in a very mild form. He took the patent remedy at a dosage of 16 pills, three times a day, and the symptoms subsided again.

One year later, there had been no recurrence of the malaria.

Manufacturer: Lanzhou Foci

Dosage: 8 pills, three times a day

Pinellia Expectorant Pills, Qing Qi Hua Tan Wan (ching chee hwah tahn wahn); "Clear Lung, Expel Phlegm Pills"

Indications: Cough due to heat, with yellow or green phlegm that is difficult to expectorate

Functions: Clears lung heat, expels phlegm, stops cough

Description: This is a standard remedy for coughs due to heat phlegm, a type of cough that occurs with heat signs, especially noted by the color of the mucus. Yellow or green phlegm that is difficult to expectorate indicates a hot phlegm condition. It is essential to use cooling, moistening expectorants to dislodge the phlegm and eliminate it from the lungs, otherwise a serious infection could develop. Originally, the pathogen (the cause of the infection, or "evil qi" in traditional terminology) is often a virus. If the person's immune system fails to repel the invader, a cold or flu results. In the course of the illness, the lungs often begin secreting large amounts of mucus. If expectorants are not employed at this point, the mucus can build up in the lungs, providing a fertile feeding ground for bacteria, resulting in an opportunistic infection (an infection that results when the immune system is weakened).

If green phlegm, indicating infection, is present, Chuan Xin Lian Antiphlogistic Pills should also be taken (3 to 6 pills, three times a day). When the mucus starts getting lighter in color and the individual is able to cough it up without difficulty, the herbs are working. As in all infections, prompt qualified medical attention is essential if symptoms worsen. In addition to herbal therapy, diet is essential in cases such as this. Sweets should be avoided, as they increase phlegm production as well as feed the infection. Light vegetable soups are easy to digest and help clear mucus, assisting the herbal formula. Do not use Pinellia Expectorant Pills for coughs due to wind cold.

Manufacturer: Lanzhou Foci

Dosage: 8 pills, three times a day

Ping Chuan Pills
(ping chwahn);
"Relieve Asthma Pills"

Indications: Chronic asthma and shortness of breath due to qi deficiency; symptoms often get worse after exertion or in the presence of a common cold

Functions: Tonifies lung and kidney qi, stops coughing, reduces phlegm

Description: This remedy is a combination of herbs with dual functions: Not only does the formula clear phlegm and calm asthma, its tonifying herbs strengthen the lungs and make them less susceptible to attacks in the future. One of the tonic herbs is *Codonopsis* (dang shen), used traditionally to strengthen the lungs and spleen (which is associated with digestive function in traditional Chinese medicine). Modern research has shown *Codonopsis* to have immune-system-strengthening properties: Its constituents stimulate the immune system and promote the production of interferon, which fights viruses and regulates the immune system. Another tonic ingredient is gecko lizard (ge jie), which strengthens the immune system. *Cordyceps*, another tonifying herb with dual functions, builds vitality and aids in the dilation (widening) of the bronchial tubes to improve breathing and help clear phlegm. The Chinese name of *Cordyceps*, dong chong xia cao, means "winter insect, summer herb." Its unusual name derives from the fact that it is a summer fungus that grows on the body of a caterpillar that died in the winter. This seemingly bizarre substance has a powerful ability to increase overall vitality. Some years ago, the Chinese women's Olympic team broke a number of swimming records; officials suspected steroid use, but all the athletes tested negative. It turns out that they were using the *Cordyceps* fungus to enhance their performance!

Manufacturer: Sing-Kyn Drug House

Dosage: 10 pills, three times a day

Yin Qiao Jie Du Pian
(yin chow jyeh doo pyen);
"Honeysuckle and Forsythia Clear-Toxin Tablets"

Indications: Acute symptoms of wind heat—sore throat, fever, headache

Functions: Expels wind heat, clears heat and toxins

Description: Along with Gan Mao Ling, this is one of the most popular Chinese patent medicines. It is highly effective in clearing wind heat types of cold or flu, for which sore throat is the cardinal symptom.

Other symptoms could be fever, intolerance for wind and cold temperatures, headache, thirst, and cough. Although most effective when taken at the onset of symptoms, this formula can also be taken during full-blown flu symptoms. Yin Qiao Jie Du Pian can also be used for pneumonia, bronchitis, tonsillitis, measles, mumps, and inner ear infections.

Classical formulas often have their chief ingredients as part of their name. The word yin, meaning silver, comes from the Chinese name for honeysuckle (jin yin hua, or gold and silver flower). The word Qiao comes from the Chinese name for forsythia (lian qiao). Honeysuckle and forsythia are often used together due to their synergistic antimicrobial effect. Clinical research shows that honeysuckle flowers and forsythia fruit inhibit the bacteria that cause pneumonia, strep throat, staphylococcal infections, salmonella, and tuberculosis. They have both been used traditionally for thousands of years to clear fire toxins, which include a hot, painful, swollen throat; boils; fevers; and urinary tract infections.

Another ingredient in Yin Qiao is *Schizonepeta* flowers (jing jie). The profuse purple flower spikes are highly aromatic, giving the herb a dispersing quality. When the body is first attacked by a pathogen, the most effective way to repel the invader is through the use of aromatic herbs that disperse their energy to the exterior of the body. The highly volatile essential oils open up the pores in the skin and act as a diaphoretic (induces sweating). If the pathogen has not penetrated to the interior of the body, this dispersing effect drives the pathogen out. Although it is warm by nature, *Schizonepeta* is effective in heat conditions when it is combined with cold herbs, as it is in this formula.

Manufacturer: Tianjin; Plum Flower. Some brands of Yin Qiao contain caffeine and over-the-counter drugs. Read the label, and make sure the patent does not contain caffeine, paracetamolum, or chlorpheniraminum.

Dosage: 4 tablets, three times a day. This remedy is for acute ailments only; do not take it for more than a few days.

Zhong Gan Ling
(jung gahn ling);
"Serious Cold Remedy"

Indications: Wind heat flu-like symptoms—high fever, sore throat

Functions: Expels wind heat, clears heat and toxins

Description: Although similar to Gan Mao Ling, Zhong Gan Ling focuses more on heat conditions. It contains gypsum (shi gao), a mineral used to clear high fevers, and Isatis (ban lang gen), a powerful antibacterial and antiviral herb, which has proved effective in treating influenza, pneumonia, meningitis, mumps, and swollen, painful throat.

Another ingredient in the formula is *Pueraria* root (ge gen), commonly known as kudzu. (This root is often used in Asian cooking as a thickening agent in sauces.) As a component of Zhong Gan Ling, kudzu has the effect of relaxing tight stiff muscles in the neck and shoulders, a common symptom of external conditions. (As a side note, recent research has shown that an extract of kudzu reduces cravings for alcohol, helping alcoholics to reduce their consumption of alcohol by 50 percent.) It is synergistic with *Notopterygium* (qiang huo), another ingredient that is effective in relieving pain in the upper body due to colds or flu.

Manufacturer: Plum Flower. It is important to use this brand only; the Meizhou brand contains Western pharmaceuticals.

Dosage: 4 to 6 pills, three times a day

Huang Lian Su Pian
(hwahng lyan soo pyen);
"Coptis Extract Tablets"

Indications: Diarrhea, infections, or dysentery due to damp heat; frequent bloody or watery stools with abdominal pain accompanied by vomiting and fever

Functions: Decreases inflammation, clears damp heat and fire toxins

Description: This formula is essential for travel to areas of the world with primitive sanitation or questionable water quality. It is remarkably effective in killing the pathogens that cause the dreaded traveler's diarrhea.

The extract is prepared from the rhizome of *Coptis chinensis* (huang lian), and the active ingredient is berberine, a powerful constituent with strong antibiotic effects. Also found in North American goldenseal and Oregon grape, berberine gives these pills their beautiful golden color.

Huang Lian Su has strong effects, inhibiting the bacteria that cause strep throat, pneumonia, and dysentery. Studies conducted in China have shown it is as effective as sulfa drugs in treating dysentery, without their serious side effects. Clinical trials have also proved it effective in treating influenza, pertussis, typhoid, tuberculosis, scarlet fever, and diphtheria. As this list of conditions illustrates, Chinese herbal medicine is highly developed and is used by practitioners to treat serious disease as well as minor ailments. This formula should not be used for diarrhea due to deficient cold conditions.

Manufacturer: Min-Kang Drug Manufactory

Dosage: 2 to 3 tablets, three times a day. This remedy is for acute conditions; it is not intended for long-term use. Do not take longer than one week.

Huo Xiang Zheng Qi Wan
(haw shahng jung chee wahn), Lophanthus Antifebrile; "Agastache Qi Normalizing Pills"

Indications: Summer damp stomach flu, with nausea, vomiting, diarrhea, sticky stools

Functions: Regulates the digestion, eliminates dampness, repels wind

Description: The chief ingredient in this formula is *Agastache* (huo xiang), also known as patchouli. This highly aromatic, easy-to-grow plant is in the category known as "aromatic herbs that transform dampness." The specific action of herbs in this category is to wake up the spleen with their strong aroma and eliminate dampness in that organ. Dampness in the spleen is characterized by symptoms of nausea, vomiting, fullness in the abdominal area, lack of appetite or thirst, and diarrhea. These symptoms usually arise as a result of acute gastroenteritis—what we often call stomach "flu"—which is effectively treated with this formula.

Highly effective, this formula often relieves symptoms with just one dose. This patent should not be taken alone in the case of fever, since it is warm by nature. When there are heat signs, such as fever, it can be taken along with Gan Mao Ling, Zhong Gan Ling, or Yin Qiao Jie Du Pien. It is best to take it for an additional day after symptoms subside to give digestive function a chance to return to normal.

Manufacturer: Lanzhou Foci

Dosage: 10 pills, three times a day

Mu Xiang Shun Qi Wan
(moo shahng shuhn chee wahn); "Saussurea Qi-Regulating Pills"

Indications: Food stagnation, indigestion, diarrhea, and flatulence

Functions: Regulates stagnant qi in the digestive organs, relieves pain in the stomach and intestines, disperses food stagnation

Description: This formula is especially effective for traveler's diarrhea and gastrointestinal discomfort when used along with Huang Lian Su. The two formulas have a powerful synergistic effect (they enhance the action of the other): The berberine in Huang Lian Su kills the pathogens that cause the digestive problem, while the carminative herbs (which relieve gas and bowel pain) in Mu Xiang Shun Qi Wan restore normal digestive function. Even in simple cases of gas or fullness, such as after eating too much or too fast, Mu Xiang Shun Qi Wan can be quite effective.

The chief ingredient in Mu Xiang Shun Qi Wan is *Saussurea lappa*, also known as *Aucklandia lappa*. This herb is very aromatic due to its high content of volatile oils, giving rise to its name, mu xiang, meaning fragrant wood. Normal function of the digestive organs requires a smooth flow of qi; stagnation of qi results in pain, distention, and abnormal activity in the organ. *Saussurea* helps promote the flow of vital energy both in the stomach and the intestines, thereby relieving pain and distention and stopping diarrhea. It acts as an antispasmodic to smooth muscle, thereby relaxing the intestines, and it inhibits the bacteria that cause dysentery.

This preparation has other positive effects in the stomach as well: It contains ginger to relieve nausea and vomiting, radish seed and hawthorn berry to move stagnant food out of the stomach, and citrus peel and barley sprouts to strengthen stomach function.

Manufacturer: Lanzhou Foci

Dosage: 8 pills, three times a day

Peach Kernel Pills, Run Chang Wan (ruhn chahng wahn); "Moisten Intestines Pills"

Indications: Constipation due to excess heat

Functions: Lubricates the intestines, promotes bowel movement, purges heat from the intestines

Description: Peach Kernel Pills act as a mild laxative, working both as an intestinal lubricant and a purgative to the large intestine when constipation due to dryness occurs. *Cannabis* seeds (huo ma ren), peach pits (tao ren), *Cistanche* (rou cong rong), and *Angelica sinensis* (dang gui) all act to lubricate the intestine, while rhubarb root (da huang) is a purgative. Therefore, this formula is best for constipation due to internal heat or dryness associated with small, hard, and difficult-to-expel stools or a burning sensation. It's important to remember that a proper diet is the key to the prevention of constipation: A person with this type of constipation should drink sufficient water and consume high fiber foods.

Manufacturer: Lanzhou Foci

Dosage: 4 to 8 pills, three times a day. The patent contains rhubarb, which stimulates the action of the bowels, so do not take this patent for more than a few days. The bowels may become dependent on any type of laxative used regularly.

Pill Curing,
Kang Ning Wan
(kahn ning wahn);
"Healthy Quiet Pills"

Indications: Disorders of the stomach, such as nausea, vomiting, fullness, acidity, motion sickness, or acid regurgitation

Functions: Regulates the digestion, calms the stomach

Description: Another very popular remedy both in China and the United States and a must for every medicine cabinet, travel kit, and purse, Pill Curing is a highly effective patent medicine. Its action centers on the stomach, where it quickly alleviates nausea, vomiting, belching, excessive stomach acid, and low appetite. It can be taken 30 to 60 minutes before travel to avoid motion sickness. In case of gastrointestinal distress accompanying the common cold, Pill Curing can be taken with Gan Mao Ling (see page 201).

Manufacturer: United Pharmaceutical Manufactory

Dosage: 1 to 2 vials, three times a day, or as needed. Each vial is filled with tiny pills; it is quite easy to wash down a whole vial of pills with water.

Sai Mei An

(sai may ahn);

"Made by Sai Mei An Factory"

Indications: Irritation to the stomach lining, gastric or duodenal ulcer without bleeding

Functions: Neutralizes excess stomach acid, stops pain, clears heat

Description: Sai Mei An treats ulcers in the stomach or duodenum, decreasing excess stomach acid, relieving pain, and coating the stomach lining. It contains the powders of a variety of shells, such as oyster or clam, giving it an acid-neutralizing, astringent effect. It also contains borneol camphor (bing pian), which helps relieve pain.

Take this remedy on an empty stomach, about half an hour before meals. It coats the stomach lining, preventing irritation of the ulcer from digestive juices and food. To continue the healing process, continue taking Sai Mei An for two weeks after symptoms subside.

Sai Mei An can also be used topically for damp skin irritations, such as poison oak or ivy rash. Its astringent ingredients help dry out the vesicles, while the camphor relieves itching. To use topically, pour the contents of one or more capsules (depending on the surface area to be treated) into the palm of the hand; slowly drip water into the powder, and mix with a finger to form a paste. Dab the paste onto the rash and allow it to dry.

Dosage: 3 capsules, three times a day

Shen Ling Bai Zhu Pian
(*shen ling buy zhoo pyen*);
"Codonopsis, Poria, and
Atractylodes Pills"

Indications: Digestive problems
due to deficient spleen, such as
loose stools, bloating, weak digestion, and belching

Functions: Tonifies spleen qi, clears
dampness, harmonizes digestion

Description: Shen Ling Bai Zhu
Pian is a reliable treatment for
chronic diarrhea or loose stools
associated with qi deficiency. In
such a pattern, the digestive dysfunction is due to internal weakness, not an infection from a virus,
bacterium, or parasite. Typically, the
symptoms develop over an extended
period and appear as indigestion,
poor appetite, loose stools or diarrhea, fatigue, and a pale face. All are
classic signs of spleen qi deficiency,
an impairment of the body's ability
to digest and absorb food. For this
reason, the components of the
patent either strengthen digestive

function and vitality or act as an
astringent to the intestines. Drawing
fluids out of the colon helps make
stools more firm.

This formula derives its name
from three major ingredients: Shen
refers to dang shen (*Codonopsis pilo-
sula*), a tonic herb often used as an
inexpensive substitute for ginseng.
In addition to improving digestion,
many herbs that tonify qi also act to
fortify the immune system. In other
words, these herbs build up the
immune system to prevent illness.
Dang shen helps the body fight off
invading pathogens that threaten the
immune system. It has also shown
an ability to increase the production
of both red and white blood cells,
which is especially significant for
chemotherapy patients. Chemotherapy destroys some disease-fighting
white blood cells in addition to cancer cells, reducing the body's ability
to fight off disease. Chemotherapy
often causes diarrhea and other
digestive system symptoms as well.
The word Ling in the name refers to

fu ling (*Poria cocos*), a wild fungus that grows around the roots of pine trees. It strengthens the spleen and harmonizes the digestive organs, assisting in fluid metabolism and promoting immune function. The words Bai Zhu refer to *Atractylodes macrocephala*, which is an aromatic qi tonic that strengthens spleen qi (the qi of digestion) and dries the damp gastrointestinal environment that leads to diarrhea. This herb also increases endurance and immune function.

Manufacturer: Plum Flower

Dosage: 6 to 12 pills, three times a day before meals

Shu Gan Wan
(shoo gahn wahn);
"Soothe Liver Pill"

Indications: Digestive disorders associated with liver imbalances, which become worse under stress; symptoms include abdominal distention and pain, nausea, belching, poor appetite, gas, and loose stools

Functions: Regulates the liver, relieves stagnation, improves digestion, relieves pain

Description: This formula is used in the condition colorfully known as "liver attacking the spleen." In this pattern, the liver is not properly functioning to allow for the smooth flow of qi. This imbalance transfers to the digestive organs, bringing on such symptoms as gas, belching, abdominal pain, indigestion, poor appetite, or loose stools. Typically, symptoms become worse when the person experiences stress. In addition to herbs that improve digestion and relieve pain and fullness, this formula contains *Bupleurum* root (chai hu), a major herb for clearing stagnation of liver function. In this way, the formula treats both the symptoms and the underlying imbalance that causes the disorder.

Manufacturer: Lanzhou Foci

Dosage: 8 pills, three times a day. Do not use during pregnancy.

Six Gentlemen Teapills,
Xiang Sha Liu Jun Wan
(shahng shah loo juhn wahn),
Aplotaxis Amomum Pills;
"Saussurea and Cardamon Six Gentlemen Pill"

Indications: Weak digestion due to spleen qi deficiency, with symptoms of poor appetite, nausea, vomiting, belching, and chronic diarrhea

Functions: Tonifies spleen qi, reduces phlegm and dampness

Description: A modern patent based on an ancient remedy, the classical formula Xiang Sha Liu Jun Zi Tang combines a qi tonic with digestive herbs. The tonic aspect of the formula consists of four herbs known as the Four Gentlemen: ginseng (ren shen), *Atractylodes* (bai zhu), *Poria* (fu ling), and Chinese licorice (zhi gan cao). These herbs make up the base of numerous formulas that treat deficiency of qi in the lungs and spleen with such chronic symptoms as fatigue, shortness of breath, pale face, lack of appetite, indigestion, and loose stools. The addition of citrus peel (chen pi) and *Pinellia* rhizome (ban xia) creates Six Gentlemen, a formula more appropriate for treating more acute cases of digestive imbalances with nausea, vomiting, and distention. The addition of *Saussurea* (mu xiang) and cardamon (sha ren) further increases the formula's ability to rectify digestive weakness and distress. It is especially appropriate for people who are pale, weak, and qi deficient with accompanying digestive weakness.

Manufacturer: Lanzhou Foci

Dosage: 8 to 16 pills, three times a day before meals

Formulas for Gynecologic Disorders

Chien Chin Chih Tai Wan
(*chyen chin chih tie wahn*);
"Thousand Gold Piece Leukorrhea Pills"

Indications: Leukorrhea (vaginal discharge)
Functions: Acts as an astringent, regulates qi, regulates blood, clears dampness
Description: This patent formula treats vaginal discharges effectively, especially in cases in which the woman has a qi deficiency marked by an overall lack of energy and vitality. It can be used for vaginal discharges, such as Trichomonas or yeast infections, especially when the discharge is light-colored. The ingredients have multiple functions: They clear the pathogen, act as an astringent to the discharge, and relieve pain.
Manufacturer: Tianjin
Dosage: 10 pills, twice a day

Xiao Yao Wan
(*shaow yaow wahn*);
"Free and Easy Wanderer Pills"

Indications: Liver qi stagnation, with irritability and menstrual imbalances
Functions: Moves stagnant liver qi; tonifies blood
Description: This classic formula could have been placed in a number of categories: It is tonifying (strengthens digestion and builds blood) and harmonizing (relieves irritability and harmonizes energy flow), and it regulates the menstrual cycle. It is by far one of the most popular patent remedies used in North America. Our high-stress lifestyle often leads to the disorder for which this formula is indicated: stagnation of qi in the liver. In traditional Chinese medicine, the liver governs the smooth flow of qi in the body and is important in regu-

lating the menstrual cycle and emotional balance. If qi is stagnant, changes in the cycle and symptoms of premenstrual syndrome occur.

Xiao Yao Wan is especially useful in cases of menstrual irregularity and discomfort as well as premenstrual syndrome and its symptoms of moodiness, breast distention, and cramping. It is most effective when used for two or three months, with a one month break afterward, then another two to three months. It should be discontinued during menstrual bleeding.

The chief herb in the formula is *Bupleurum* root (chai hu), a very important plant in Chinese medicine. *Bupleurum* is well-known for its ability to stimulate the immune system, suppress flu viruses, and bring down fevers. It is also anti-inflammatory and has a tranquilizing effect. It is the chief herb for treating disorders of the liver, especially when stagnant qi leads to emotional irritability.

Manufacturer: Lanzhou Foci

Dosage: 8 to 10 pills, three times daily

Yu Dai Wan
(yoo dye wahn);
"Heal Leukorrhea Pills"

Indications: Leukorrhea (vaginal discharge) due to damp heat

Functions: Clears damp heat in the lower burner

Description: Yu Dai Wan is another effective treatment for vaginal discharge. Unlike Chien Chin, which is appropriate for both heat and cold conditions, Yu Dai Wan is specific for discharges due to heat. The main indicator for a heat-type discharge is a yellow or dark color with a strong smell. This is considered a condition of damp heat: The discharge is a form of dampness, and the yellow color and strong smell are signs of heat. Therefore, the treatment principle is to drain the dampness and clear the heat. This is accomplished through the cold, astringent action of the formula's chief herb, *Ailanthus altissima* (chun pi). The cold nature of the herb helps clear the heat, while its astringent action helps dry the discharge. In addition to nourishing herbs that assist the body's "cooling system" (yin), the formula also contains *Phellodendron* bark (huang bai), a powerful antibiotic herb that has shown great success in treating vaginitis and cervicitis from trichomonas infections. **Warning:** Do not confuse this herb with philodendron, a common, poisonous houseplant.

Manufacturer: Lanzhou Foci

Dosage: 8 to 10 pills, three times a day

Chin Koo Tieh Shang Wan
(*chin koo dyeh shahng wahn*);
"Muscles and Bones
Injury Pill"

Indications: Traumatic injuries,
bruises, sprains, and swelling
Functions: Moves blood, reduces
swelling and internal bleeding,
relieves pain
Description: Chin Koo Tieh Shang
Wan is useful for traumatic injuries
that have bruising and swelling as
the primary symptoms. The chief
herb in the formula is *Panax pseudoginseng* (san qi), which is also the
active ingredient in Yunnan Pai Yao.
Chin Koo also contains myrrh (mo
yao) and frankincense (ru xiang),
two herbs that are commonly paired
to increase circulation and reduce
pain. These same herbs have also
been used as incense for thousands
of years. The essential oils that give
them their heavenly aroma also act
to stimulate blood circulation. Since
traditional Chinese medicine sees
stagnation of qi and blood as the
major cause of pain, circulatory
stimulants are the treatment of
choice in traumatic injuries.
Manufacturer: Tientsin Drug Manufactory
Dosage: 10 pills, three times a day
until injury improves

Du Huo Ji Sheng Wan
(*doo hwaw jee shuhng wahn*);
"Angelica Loranthus Pills"

Indications: Cold, damp type pain
and stiffness in the low back and
knees with underlying deficiency of
qi and blood
Functions: Expels wind dampness,
relieves pain, tonifies the liver and
kidneys
Description: This is another classic
formula, first put into writing about
1,200 years ago. A very elegant and

subtle formulation, it not only relieves pain, it also strengthens any underlying deficiencies that make one susceptible to injury. The specific indications for the formula are pain in the lower back and knees accompanied by general weakness, stiffness, and a desire for warmth, especially in the areas of pain. While especially appropriate for the elderly due to its tonifying and strengthening qualities, it is useful for anybody with arthritis, chronic low back pain, or sciatica.

The formula derives its name from two of the principal ingredients, du huo (*Angelica pubescens*) and sang ji sheng (*Loranthus parasiticus*). Du huo is specific for rheumatic pain that is sensitive to cold, especially if it occurs in the lower body. Its pharmaceutical actions are antirheumatic, anti-inflammatory, and analgesic (pain relieving). Sang ji sheng has dual functions: It strengthens the liver and kidneys while subsequently nourishing the bones and tendons, and it relieves the pain of arthritis. As a "side effect," it lowers blood pressure and is useful in coronary heart disease. Other ingredients in the formula include the basic formulas to tonify both qi and blood, which assist the remedy in returning strength, vitality, and strong immune function, making it especially useful for long-term use by elderly or weakened patients.

Du Huo Ji Sheng Wan is a very popular formula, with a well-deserved reputation for bringing relief to chronic pain due to cold and dampness.

Manufacturer: Min Kang Pharmaceutical Manufactory

Dosage: 6 pills, three times a day

Sciatica Pills

Indications: Sciatic pain

Functions: Stimulates blood circulation, relieves pain

Description: These pills effectively treat sciatica, a painful condition that follows the course of the sciatic nerve. Typically, the pain is caused by compression of a nerve by a protruding disk; often, the pain travels through the buttocks and down the back of the leg. In addition to Sciatica Pills, acupuncture is often very effective in treating this condition.

Some cases of sciatic pain respond to one acupuncture treatment and a short course of herbal therapy, while others are exceptionally resistant to recovery. The outcome depends on a number of factors: the overall health of the person, the severity of the injury causing the sciatic pain, and the ability of the person to rest and allow healing to occur. Sciatica Pills work especially well when combined with Du Huo Ji Sheng Wan.

Manufacturer: Hongxing Pharmaceutical Manufactory

Dosage: 10 pills, three times a day. Take for 15 days.

Specific Lumbaglin,
Te Xiao Yao Tong Pian
(teh shaow yaow tuhng pyen);
"Effective Low Back Pain Pills"

Indications: Lower back pain, muscle strains, sciatic pain

Functions: Expels wind dampness, relieves pain and inflammation, tonifies yang

Description: This remedy is similar to Du Huo Ji Sheng Wan, but it is more specific for low back pain due to injuries. It comes in a blister pack of capsules that's great for a travel kit. It relieves low back pain quickly in all but the most stubborn cases.

Manufacturer: Guangzhou Pharmaceutical Industrial Corporation

Dosage: 1 to 2 capsules, three times a day

Yan Hu Suo Zhi Tong Pian
(yahn hoo swaw jih tuhng pyen);
"Corydalis Stop Pain Tablets"

Indications: Pain that is due to qi and blood stagnation, menstrual pain, abdominal pain, pain from injuries

Functions: Invigorates blood, relieves pain, relaxes muscle spasms

Description: This formula comes in two varieties; one is an herbal extract, the other is a pharmaceutical extract. The label shows a subtle difference: the pharmaceutical extract is called Yan Hu Su, while the herbal extract is called Yan Hu Suo. The herbal extract also lists *Angelica* root as an ingredient. While the pharmaceutical extract is stronger, it is essentially a drug, so choose the natural herbal extract. This remedy helps relieve pain of menstrual discomfort, liver or gallbladder problems, angina, muscle spasms, or injuries. It can have a tranquilizing effect, making it useful for treating insomnia due to pain. Because it can cause drowsiness in some people, it should not be used when driving.

The active ingredient in this formula is *Corydalis* tuber (yan hu suo), a powerful sedative and analgesic. Its pain-relieving effect is consid-

ered to be about one percent that of opium.

Manufacturer: Chongqing

Dosage: 4 pills, three times a day

Yunnan Pai Yao (*yuhnahn pie yow*); "White Medicine from Yunnan"

Indications: External and internal bleeding from a variety of causes

Functions: Controls bleeding and bruising, reduces swelling, relieves pain

Description: This patent medicine is one of the miracles of Chinese herbal medicine: Its ability to stop bleeding and reduce swelling and pain are legendary. During the war in Vietnam, dead Vietcong soldiers were often found with a small vial of Yunnan Pai Yao hanging around their necks. They sprinkled it on gunshot wounds to stop the bleeding while they waited to be evacuated for medical treatment. Its effects are so powerful, it can stop bleeding from stomach ulcers or cancer, hemophilia, and severe injuries. In case of excessive blood loss, a small red pill is included with each package to prevent the person from going into shock. The red pill should not be taken unless severe loss of blood has occurred and the person is losing consciousness. Of course, these are all serious conditions requiring immediate medical care.

In addition to its usefulness in life-threatening conditions, Yunnan Pai Yao is remarkable in its ability to stop swelling and pain due to sports injuries and accidents.

Although the exact formulation of this patent is considered a family secret, it is almost 100 percent *Panax pseudoginseng* (san qi). This herb is a close relative of Asian ginseng (*Panax ginseng*) and American ginseng (*Panax quinquefolium*). However, san qi is used primarily for injuries, while the others are used to build vitality and immunity. In more than 50 years of scientific study, *Panax pseudoginseng* has been shown to have significant benefits. It can decrease clotting time for blood, a significant benefit to people with clotting disorders.

Yunnan Pai Yao can also be used topically to stop bleeding. Wash the injured area thoroughly with water and apply the patent directly to the injury. Apply pressure, then bandage the area. For deeper wounds, squeeze the cut together before pouring on the powder and hold it shut for a few minutes. It is important to see a doctor immediately afterward in case the cut requires stitches.

Manufacturer: Yunnan Pai Yao Factory

Dosage: 1 to 2 capsules, three or four times a day

Topical Formulas for Injuries

701 Plasters and Hua Tuo Plasters

(hwah twaw)

Indications: Pain from sprains, traumatic injuries, or muscular tension

Functions: Stimulates circulation, relieves pain

Description: Packaged as four adhesive squares, 701 Plasters are coated with highly aromatic herbs that assist in blood circulation and pain relief. To use, peel off the plastic backing sheet and place the plaster over the sore area. Within a few minutes, you will feel warmth in the area, which disappears a short time later. The pain-relieving effects last about 24 hours, after which you peel off the plaster and discard it. It is best to wait a few hours before applying another plaster, since some people can experience mild irritation from them.

These patches are very effective for soreness due to muscle strains or injuries; however, never apply them over skin that is broken. When using them to treat muscle tightness, especially in the upper back and shoulders where people typically store tension, it is important to apply them bilaterally, even if only one side is sore. If the patch is applied to one side only, it is very common for the pain to move to the opposite side! From the perspective of traditional Chinese medicine, this phenomenon is easily explained. Pain that comes and goes, such as muscle tension, is considered a condition of wind. By its nature, wind comes and goes unpredictably; it also can appear in different places without warning. Since the nature of the plaster is to disperse wind, it is important to ensure it does not have any place to reappear.

Hua Tuo plasters are nearly the same as 701 Plasters; the only real difference is they stick more tenaciously to the skin. For this reason, they are more appropriate for areas that flex, such as joints. Because 701 Plasters don't stick quite as well, they are ideal for hair-covered areas; removing them causes very little pain from hair pulled by the adhesive.

Manufacturer: Guangzhou Medicines & Health Products

Ching Wan Hung,
Jing Wan Hong
(*ching wahn huhng*);
"Capital Absolute Red"

Indications: Burns of all kinds
Functions: Clears heat, relieves pain, promotes healing
Description: Without a doubt, this miracle cream has a welcome place in any first-aid kit. Its ability to heal burns quickly is almost beyond belief. It can be applied to first and second degree burns as long as

there is no infection. As soon as the ointment comes in contact with the skin, the pain begins to recede. In China, it is used for burns caused by hot water or steam, chemicals, radiation, and sunburn. Apply the cream, then cover the burn with a dressing, which you should change daily. For simple first degree burns, no dressing is necessary. Be aware that this salve stains clothing.

Manufacturer: Tianjin

Zheng Gu Shui
(*juhng goo shway*);
"Setting Bone Liquid"

Indications: Traumatic injuries, bruises, sprains
Functions: Relieves blood stagnation, promotes healing, stops pain
Description: This highly effective liniment can be used for all sorts of injuries; however, its specialty is to reduce pain and promote healing of broken bones. If the skin is not broken, it can be applied topically to the area of injury to relieve pain

until the bone is set at the hospital. For sprains and sports injuries, it can be applied at any time. Similar effective liniments are Po Sum On Medicated Oil and Tieh Ta Yao Gin. If the skin is broken or burned at the site of the injury, use Wan Hua Oil, which is safe to apply in these conditions.

Caution: Do not use on open wounds. Some people experience a skin reaction from liniments; discontinue use immediately if a reaction develops. Avoid exposing the treated area to sun to avoid irritation. Wash hands thoroughly after applying. This patent is for external use only. Keep tightly closed and out of reach of children. Do not use Zheng Gu Shui near an open flame as it is flammable. This liniment stains clothing.

Manufacturer: Yulin Drug Manufactory

Formulas for Reducing Inflammation

Fargelin for Piles (High Strength),
Qiang Li Hua Zhi Ling
(chyahng lee hwah jih ling);
"Extra Strength Effective Eliminate Hemorrhoids"

Indications: Acute and chronic hemorrhoids
Functions: Invigorates blood, relieves pain, reduces swelling, clears heat
Description: Add this remedy to the list of remarkable Chinese medicines. People frequently report overnight relief from the pain, swelling, and bleeding of hemorrhoids. **Note:** The label lists bear gallbladder as one of the ingredients. Typically, this ingredient has been replaced by the gallbladder of a domestic animal, or the patent contains no animal products. Continued international pressure should ensure that the Chinese discontinue

the practice of using body parts from endangered species.
Manufacturer: United Drug Manufactory
Dosage: 3 tablets, taken three times a day

Lian Qiao Bai Du Pian
(lyahn chow bye doo pyen);
"Forsythia Clear Toxins Tablets"

Indications: Skin inflammations and infections
Functions: Clears heat and inflammation, relieves pain
Description: Lian Qiao Bai Du Pian is a useful formula for treating a wide variety of skin eruptions due to toxic heat, such as boils, skin infections, and poison oak or ivy. In all cases of skin inflammation, it is essential to make adjustments in the diet as well. One way the body eliminates irritating or unhealthy substances is through the skin. A

diet that is high in irritating substances such as coffee and spicy and greasy foods, therefore, often leads to skin problems. In fact, coffee is so heating to the blood that it can be almost impossible to clear an individual's skin problems as long as he or she continues to drink it. Since this heat in the blood is a result of an internal process, it is very difficult to resolve skin eruptions or skin inflammation with the application of topical creams or ointments. However, when blood-cooling herbs are taken internally, the inflammation is dealt with at the source.

In one case, a young woman had been suffering for weeks from severe poison oak. Her thigh was swollen, stiff, and bright red; even a cortisone shot failed to relieve the symptoms. She was given a bulk herbal formula similar to Lian Qiao Bai Du Pian to drink three times a day; an external wash consisting of astringent herbs was also applied to relieve the itching and to help dry

up the rash. In addition, her diet was adjusted to include cooling foods such as salads and carrot juice. After one week, her leg had returned to normal. She continued on a maintenance dose of the patent medicine for another week to make sure that the inflammation was gone, and she eliminated coffee from her diet.

Lian Qiao Bai Du Pian contains rhubarb root (da huang), which helps to clear toxic heat. It accomplishes this by increasing bowel movements. This purgative effect should be considered before taking the remedy.

Manufacturer: Tianjin

Dosage: 4 to 6 pills, three times a day

Long Dan Xie Gan Wan (luhng dahn shyeh gahn wahn); "Gentian Clear the Liver Pills"

Indications: Excess heat in the liver causing conjunctivitis, urinary tract infection, prostatitis

Functions: Clears damp heat and fire from the liver and from the gallbladder

Description: This traditional formula treats a wide range of inflammatory conditions. Its actions are most easily understood when considered from the perspective of traditional Chinese disease patterns. This patent is indicated strictly for excess-type disorders rather than deficiency-type conditions. While deficiency conditions require a strengthening or tonifying of the body, in conditions of excess, the proper treatment is often to clear heat or drain dampness. Long Dan Xie Gan Wan is specific for the patterns known as excess heat or damp heat in the liver and gallbladder, with symptoms that include red eyes, headache, bitter taste in the mouth, irritability, and possible hearing loss. Other symptoms of "lower burner damp heat" are dark or cloudy urine, genital itching or swelling, vaginal discharge, and constipation.

The numerous imbalances Long Dan Xie Gan Wan is able to resolve are organized by organ system as follows:

- Eyes: acute conjunctivitis ("pink eye"), corneal ulcers, acute glaucoma, retinitis
- Ears: acute middle ear infection, acute external ear infection
- Urinary: acute urinary tract infection (kidney, bladder, or urethra)
- Reproductive: genital herpes, pelvic inflammatory disease, vaginal discharge, testicular swelling or inflammation, acute prostatitis
- Systemic: migraine, eczema, herpes zoster
- Liver and Gallbladder: acute hepatitis, acute cholecystitis

Although the medical conditions listed above appear unrelated, they can share the same traditional Chinese diagnosis. For this reason, it is essential to treat the individual's traditional symptom patterns, not the

Western disease name. Just as a single Chinese diagnostic category can manifest as numerous and widely different Western diseases, a single Western disease can also have a wide range of Chinese diagnoses, depending on an individual's symptoms and constitution.

In one memorable case in which Long Dan Xie Gan Wan was effective, a patient had severe conjunctivitis in one eye for a few weeks. She had already gone through a round of antibiotics with no resolution, and she was beginning to feel desperate. Her symptom pattern fit the diagnosis of excess heat in the liver, so she was given Long Dan Xie Gan Wan. In addition, a tea of chrysanthemum flowers (ju hua) was prescribed to reduce inflammation specifically in the eye. After one week of Chinese herbal therapy, the eye returned to normal. At this point, the condition of excess heat was cleared, and it was time to address the underlying weakness, a deficiency of liver yin. When the

moistening, cooling, yin aspect of the liver is deficient, the organ tends to overheat, making it more prone to inflammation. For example, if a car engine is low on oil or water (yin) it has a tendency to overheat. Once it overheats, the first step is to let it cool down (clear excess heat). To address the cause of the overheating, oil and water are added (tonifying yin). In this way, traditional Chinese medicine is very thorough in its treatment of disease; it not only corrects the problem but resolves the cause as well.

In another case, Long Dan Xie Gan Wan was used to treat an attack of genital herpes in a young woman. As is often the case with outbreaks of the herpesvirus, the young woman could sense the attack coming on before actual symptoms appeared, giving her a chance to begin treatment before the full-blown manifestation. Since the symptoms fit the pattern of damp heat in the liver meridian, she immediately began a course of Long

Dan Xie Gan Wan along with acupuncture therapy. The outbreak was not only milder than usual but it went into remission very quickly compared with her previous outbreaks.

Manufacturer: Lanzhou Foci

Dosage: 8 pills, three times a day. This patent should be discontinued as soon as symptoms subside since long-term use can weaken digestion.

Prostate Gland Pills,
Qian Lie Xian Wan
(chyahn lyeh shahn wahn)

Indications: Acute and chronic prostatitis, testicular pain

Functions: Clears damp heat in the lower burner, stimulates circulation, decreases inflammation

Description: As the name implies, this remedy is formulated for acute or chronic inflammation of the prostate gland. This disorder is especially common in males older than 40 years of age. Symptoms include dribbling or painful urination and pain in the testicles. The remedy is also useful for urinary tract infections and testicular inflammation. In two cases of testicular pain due to trauma, one in a marathon runner and the other in a bicycle racer, a course of Prostate Gland Pills along with some rest from their athletic activity was all they needed. Treatment took only a week. Chronic cases of inflammation may require a longer course of treatment.

The chief herb in the formula is *Vaccaria* seed (wang bu liu xing), which is useful for painful swellings in the breasts or testicles.

Note: Prostate cancer is very common in older men; anyone experiencing prostate problems should consult his physician and undergo diagnostic testing for the disease.

Manufacturer: Wai Yeung District Medicine Company

Dosage: 6 pills, three times a day

Bu Zhong Yi Qi Wan
(*boo juhng yee chee wahn*),
Central Chi Tea;
**"Tonify the Middle,
Strengthen Qi Pills"**

Indications: Qi deficiency, weak
digestion, prolapsed organs, fatigue

Functions: Tonifies qi, regulates
digestion, raises yang (pulls up prolapsed organs)

Description: An ancient formula,
Bu Zhong Yi Qi Wan has a long history of resolving digestive problems
and prolapsed organs, both conditions due to qi deficiency. Although
primarily composed of tonifying
herbs, this formula also contains
two herbs that perform a task
unique to Chinese medicine. Cimicifuga (sheng ma) and *Bupleurum*
(chai hu) are used as directing
herbs with an upward energy; that
is, in addition to their specific medicinal effects, they can also direct

the effects of an herb formula to the
upper portion of the body. This
upward energy can also be
employed to resolve organ prolapse,
a condition in which an organ, such
as the uterus, bladder, or rectum,
sags downward due to connective
tissue weakness. The formula is also
useful—when prescribed and
supervised by an experienced practitioner—for the condition known
in Western medicine as "incompe-
tent uterus" in which miscarriage
occurs between the third and sixth
months of pregnancy due to cervical weakness. In addition to
strengthening prolapsed organs, Bu
Zhong Yi Qi Wan can be used for
other symptoms of spleen and
stomach qi deficiency, such as
fatigue, abdominal bloating, sensitivity to cold, and chronic diarrhea.

Manufacturer: Lanzhou Foci

Dosage: 8 pills, three times a day

Extractum Astragali,
Bei Qi Jing
(bay chee jing);
"Essence of Northern
Astragalus"

Indications: Fatigue, weak immune system

Functions: Tonifies spleen qi and lung qi

Description: Available in small one-dose vials, this remedy is a 50/50 mixture of honey and *Astragalus* root (huang qi). This perennial member of the pea family produces a large yellow root that is highly prized in Chinese herbal medicine. It is often cooked in soup bases to provide a boost to the vital energy. A safe and effective herb, it strengthens the immune system (wei qi) by increasing production of antibodies and macrophages, cells that attack disease-causing pathogens and foreign objects in the body. It is also used to strengthen spleen qi, meaning it improves digestive function and overall vitality. It helps nourish the blood and "generate flesh," making it useful for skin ulcers that won't heal and postsurgical recovery. In China, it is routinely given to women who have undergone surgery to remove fibroid tumors from the uterus. This operation frequently leaves the uterine wall in a thin, weakened state, making future pregnancies a risk. *Astragalus* is used to help surgical patients grow new muscle tissue in the uterus before scarring sets in.

The blood-building aspect of this herb can be seen in its use after chemotherapy, a procedure that causes severe disruptions in white blood cell count. Combined in a decoction with *Ligustrum* seeds (nu zhen zi), this remedy has been found to normalize the blood count.

Manufacturer: Changchun

Dosage: 1 to 2 vials per day

Ginseng Royal Jelly Vials,
Ren Shen Feng Wang Jiang
(ren shen fuhng wahng jyahng);
"Ginseng and
Royal Jelly Syrup"

Indications: Fatigue, poor appetite, feeling cold and weak

Functions: Tonifies qi and yang

Description: Asian ginseng is a strong tonic to several organ systems. With its warm energy, it is especially appropriate for weak, cold individuals who have both qi deficiency and yang deficiency. Symptoms of this deficiency condition include fatigue, low immunity, pale face and tongue, and feeling cold all the time. It has a significant ability to reduce fatigue and strengthen the immune system. Because of its warm nature, Asian ginseng is not recommended for individuals with high blood pressure or a high metabolism with a tendency to overheat. For these individuals, American ginseng (*Panax quinquefolium*), with its cool-ing, moist, yin-enhancing nature, is more appropriate.

At one time considered an exotic curiosity from Asia, ginseng products such as this are now sold all over North America. It's not uncommon to find these vials sitting at cash registers at the most unlikely of places, such as convenience or liquor stores. Although the syrup contains very little ginseng, it is still quite effective at building overall energy. For more serious tonification, a stronger extract is recommended, such as the liquid Panax Ginseng Extractum or the thick syrup, "Pure Concentrated Korean Red Ginseng Tea." To truly experience the power of ginseng, there is no substitute for boiling a whole root for an hour or two and drinking the liquid.

The amount of research conducted on the effects of ginseng is staggering. Ginseng root has been found to enhance the ability of the nervous system to adapt to stress, stabilize blood pressure in cases of shock, and have a synergistic effect with insulin, which may allow a person with diabetes to reduce the amount of insulin used to control blood sugar levels.

Manufacturer: China National Native Products

Dosage: 1 to 2 vials a day

Kwei Be Wan, Gui Pi Wan (*gway pee wahn*), *Angelica Longana Tea*, "Bring Back the Spleen Pills"

Indications: Fatigue, palpitations, poor memory, insomnia

Functions: Tonifies spleen qi and heart blood

Description: This ancient classical formula, available in convenient pill form, treats symptoms of deficiency in both the heart and spleen. This sort of imbalance often arises as a result of excessive thinking or preoccupation and is often referred to as "student's syndrome." Symptoms of spleen qi deficiency include fatigue, poor digestion, abdominal distention, loose stools, and pale face. The ingredients used to fortify the spleen are *Codonopsis* (dang shen), *Poria* (fu ling), *Saussurea* (mu xiang), *Atractylodes* (bai zhu), licorice (gan cao), and *Astragalus* (huang qi). The symptoms of heart blood deficiency are insomnia, poor memory, restless dreaming, mental restlessness, and dizziness. These are addressed by the inclusion of *Ziziphus* seed (suan zao ren), *Polygala* (yuan zhi), *Angelica sinensis* (dang gui), and longan fruit (long yan rou). Since a deficiency of spleen qi involves an impairment of the body's ability to assimilate nutrients through digestion, it often leads to a deficiency of blood. Therefore, the qi tonic herbs synergistically assist the blood tonic herbs in enriching the heart blood, another demonstration of the subtle elegance of traditional Chinese herbal medicine.

Manufacturer: Lanzhou Foci

Dosage: 8 pills, three times a day

Ming Mu Di Huang Wan (*ming moo dee hwahng wahn*); "Brighten Eyes Rehmannia Pills"

Indications: Dry eyes, blurry vision, poor eyesight, all due to underlying yin deficiency

Functions: Tonifies liver and kidney yin, nourishes the eyes

Description: One of the variations of the Liu Wei Di Huang Wan base formula, this remedy adds three ingredients to focus the actions on the eyes. The first addition is *Lycium* fruit (gou qi zi), a delicious reddish raisinlike berry that can be eaten fresh. It is used in formulas where the liver and kidneys lack sufficient yin or blood to nourish the eyes. In clinical studies, *Lycium* berries have been found to have a protective effect on the liver. Since the liver is the major organ responsible for detoxifying harmful substances in the body, it can suffer damage from some of these toxins. *Lycium* fruit can reduce damage to liver cells and speed recovery of normal liver function.

The other two additions to the base formula are abalone shell (shi jue ming) and *Tribulus* fruit (bai ji li)—both are specific for eye problems caused by a disturbance in the liver (liver heat or liver wind). The entire formula is, therefore, quite useful for eye problems due to an underlying deficiency of liver and kidney yin. It can be used for poor visual acuity, night blindness, sensitivity to light (photophobia), excessive tearing, or retinitis. It is important to be sure of an underlying yin deficiency; if the condition is one of excess fire (acute, swollen, red inflamed eyes), formulas that clear heat should be used, such as Long Dan Xie Gan Wan.

Manufacturer: Lanzhou Foci

Dosage: 8 to 10 pills, three times a day

Nu Ke Ba Zhen Wan
(noo keh bah jen wahn),
Women's Precious Pills;
"Gynecology Eight
Treasure Pills"

Indications: Fatigue, dizziness, anemia, scanty menses, lack of appetite

Functions: Tonifies qi and blood

Description: Derived from a 13th century formula, this remedy is a combination of two other classic formulas; one is a qi tonic, the other, a blood tonic. The base formula to strengthen qi is known as Four Gentlemen (Si Jun Zi Tang) and comprises ginseng (ren shen), *Atractylodes* (bai zhu), *Poria* (fu ling), and honey-fried licorice (zhi gan cao). (Frequently, Codonopsis [dang shen] replaces ginseng as a cheaper, less heating alternative.) The base formula to tonify blood is known as Four Substances (Si Wu Tang); it contains prepared *Rehmannia* (shu di huang), *Angelica sinensis* (dang gui), *Paeonia* root (bai shao), and *Ligusticum* (chuan xiong). The combination of these two classics in this remedy makes it appropriate for a generalized deficiency of both qi and blood, so it is especially useful for women because of their monthly loss of blood during menstruation. It should be taken only after bleeding has subsided, not during the menstrual period.

Symptoms of deficiency of qi and blood include fatigue, pale face, dizziness, heart palpitations, shortness of breath, and poor appetite. Other signs include irregular menstruation, painful menstruation, slight or no menstrual flow, and weakness during pregnancy or the postpartum period. Clinical research on this formula in China demonstrated that this combination of herbs normalizes the blood count in cases of acute anemia.

Manufacturer: Lanzhou Foci

Dosage: 8 to 10 pills, three times a day

Rehmannia Teapills,
Liu Wei Di Huang Wan
(loo way dee hwahng wahn),
Six Flavor Tea; "Six Ingredient Rehmannia Pills"

Indications: Thirst, irritability, night sweats, insomnia, weak low back and knees

Functions: Tonifies kidney yin, clears heat from yin deficiency conditions

Description: This is the classical base formula for all conditions of yin deficiency, especially of the liver and kidneys. Yin is moist, cool, and calm, and it enriches the organs and acts as a lubricant to bodily functions. When yin is deficient, chronic dryness and inflammation can occur. Yin deficiency can be compared with running a car that is low on oil: Under normal operating conditions, the lack of lubrication causes the engine to run hotter than normal; continued operation under these conditions can lead to long-term damage.

A variety of factors can cause yin to become deficient, such as overwork, lack of sufficient rest, insufficient fluid intake, stress, an overly dry environment, and excessive sexual activity. Symptoms of liver and kidney yin deficiency include a warm sensation in the sternum, palms, and soles of the feet; red cheeks; night sweats; a feeling of heat and irritability in the afternoon and evening; sore and weak low back and knees; ringing in the ears; chronic dry mouth; thirst; a reddish tongue with little or no coating; and a thin, rapid pulse. By focusing on nourishing yin and clearing the heat from the deficiency, this formula subtly and elegantly treats this wide range of seemingly unrelated symptoms. It contains three ingredients that nourish yin and three that clear the deficiency heat.

The chief tonifying herb in the formula is *Rehmannia glutinosa* (di huang), an extremely important herb in the *Materia Medica* (see page 12). In its raw state, it has a cold energy and is used to clear heat and nourish yin, making it useful in the treatment of high fevers and thirst due to diabetes. The prepared form is treated with wine to make it more nourishing to the blood and is used to treat anemia and menstrual difficulties and as an overall tonic to the kidneys and adrenal glands.

Another important ingredient in Rehmannia Teapills is *Dioscorea*, or Chinese yam (shan yao), a tonic to the lungs, stomach, and kidneys. It also induces the production of interferon, a substance manufactured by the immune system; interferon prevents viruses from replicating without disturbing normal cell function. The third tonic herb is *Cornus officinalis*, or dogwood fruit (shan zhu yu), an astringent herb with a variety of actions: It is antiallergic, diuretic, antihypertensive, antitumor, antibacterial, and antifungal, and it increases the production of white blood cells. An astringent, it prevents further depletion of yin, preventing the excessive loss of semen, perspiration, urine, and uterine blood.

Another ingredient, *Alisma plantago*, or water plantain (ze xie), a strong diuretic and antibacterial herb, lowers blood pressure, cholesterol, and blood sugar, another reason this formula is so effective in controlling diabetes. A sedating herb included in the formula is *Poria cocos* (fu ling), a diuretic herb that also has a calming effect on the body. It is one of the important herbs for stimulating the immune system; it induces interferon production and contains polysaccharides that stimulate the immune system to track down and destroy cells foreign to the body. The final herb in the formula is moutan, or tree peony root bark (mu dan pi), an aromatic agent that cools the body on a number of levels. It kills *Staphylococcus* organisms, lowers blood pressure, and decreases body temperature.

Liu Wei Di Huang Wan is a highly sophisticated formula that is useful in a wide variety of conditions. Numerous modifications to this base formula are available for specific conditions. Some of the disorders Liu Wei Di Huang Wan treats are diabetes, tuberculosis, hyperthyroidism, nephritis, hypertension, chronic urinary tract infection, and various degenerative diseases of the eyes. With some conditions, such as tuberculosis, Western pharmaceuticals are taken along with the herbs.

Note: Many of these conditions are life-threatening. As with all of the remedies in this book, the care of a qualified physician is essential while working with the herbs.

Manufacturer: Lanzhou Foci

Dosage: 8 to 16 pills, three times a day. Since this is a tonic formula, it should be taken for a few months.

Shen Qi Da Bu Wan
(shen chee dah boo wahn);
"Codonopsis Astragalus Great Tonifying Pill"

Indications: Weak immunity, fatigue, lack of appetite

Functions: Tonifies lung and spleen qi, strengthens immunity.

Description: Shen Qi Da Bu Wan is a general tonic for qi, blood, and immune function (wei qi). It is a mixture of *Astragalus* (see description under Extractum Astragali) and *Codonopsis* root (dang shen). Both herbs are important tonics, and combined they make a balanced formula. They have a synergistic effect, since they both stimulate the central nervous system, lower blood pressure, stimulate the immune system, and increase the blood count.

Manufacturer: Lanzhou Foci

Dosage: 8 to 10 pills, three times a day

Shou Wu Chih
(show woo cherh);
"Polygonum He Shou Wu Juice"

Indications: Fatigue, poor vision, general debility, premature aging

Functions: Tonifies blood and essence

Description: Shou Wu Chih is another convenient liquid tonic. The chief herb is *Polygonum multiflorum* (he shou wu), also incorrectly known as fo ti. Essentially a blood tonic, he shou wu nourishes liver and kidney essence, treating such conditions as weakness, insomnia, blurred vision, and premature graying of the hair. The herb's name is due to an old tale about its discovery. As the story goes, Mr. He was an old, gray-haired man who went off into the hills to die so he would not become a burden to his family. After a few months, he wandered back into his village looking quite healthy with a full head of black hair. When questioned about how he managed to thrive so well in the wild, he replied that he had survived by eating the roots of a wild vine, *Polygonum multiflorum*. Since then, the plant has been known as he shou wu, or "black-haired Mr. He." In addition to its nourishing quality, he shou wu has demonstrated effectiveness in lowering blood cholesterol levels and inhibiting the pathogens that cause tuberculosis and malaria.

In addition to other yin and blood tonics such as *Angelica sinensis* (dang gui) and *Rehmannia glutinosa* (shu di huang), the formula also contains small quantities of cloves (ding xiang, or "fragrant spike") and cardamon (sha ren). The inclusion of these aromatic carminative herbs makes the formula more digestible. Tonic herbs, even those meant to strengthen digestive function, are often heavy and difficult to digest. For this reason, digestive stimulants are often added to tonic formulas to prevent digestive discomfort.

Manufacturer: United Drug Manufactory

Dosage: 2 to 3 tablespoons mixed with water or tea, three times a day. The remedy can be taken over a long period if the individual has no heat signs (red face, dry mouth, irritability, skin rash).

Tang Kwei Gin
(*dahng gway jin*);
"Angelica Dang Gui Syrup"

Indications: Fatigue, anemia, scanty menses

Functions: Tonifies qi and blood, regulates menses

Description: A classic blood tonic, Tang Kwei Gin comes in a liquid form that is quite pleasant-tasting when mixed in water. When used along with Women's Precious Pills, it can raise the red blood cell count, an important action in cases of anemia or fatigue after surgery or a prolonged illness. It also strengthens digestive function, helping the body absorb nutrients from food and further assisting in the production of new blood cells.

The chief herb in the formula is *Angelica sinensis* (dang gui), a sweetly aromatic root with a wide range of actions. It has a regulatory effect on the uterus, enabling contractions to be more regular (such as in cases of delayed or weak menstruation) or relaxing the uterine muscle (such as with cramps), depending on which is needed. The formula also contains vitamin B12, which is necessary to prevent pernicious anemia.

Manufacturer: Plum Flower

Dosage: 1 tablespoon, three times a day

Zhi Bai Di Huang Wan
(*jih bye dee hwahng wahn*),
Chih Pai Ti Huang Wan;
"Anemarrhena and Phellodendron with Rehmannia Pills"

Indications: Hot flashes, night sweats, irritability, menopausal symptoms, all due to strong heat arising from yin deficiency

Functions: Tonifies yin and clears heat from yin deficiency conditions

Description: This variation on Liu Wei Di Huang Wan has two added ingredients: *Anemarrhena* root (zhi mu) and *Phellodendron* bark (huang bai). The addition of these two heat-clearing herbs makes the formula much colder, enhancing its ability to clear heat from deficiency of yin. This makes it more useful than the base formula, Liu Wei Di Huang Wan, when deficiency heat is the major symptom as in night sweats, hot flashes, thirst, restlessness, red cheeks, and dark urine. It is very useful in treating the symptoms of menopause, where the deficiency of yin (estrogen) leads to deficiency heat (hot flashes, night sweats, restlessness). It is also effective in treating the same symptoms in people who have developed deficiency heat signs after long-term use of thyroid replacement hormones or lithium.

Manufacturer: Lanzhou Foci

Dosage: 8 to 16 pills, three times a day

An Mien Pien

(ahn myehn pyen);
"Peaceful Sleep Tablets"

Indications: Insomnia, anxiety,
poor memory

Functions: Nourishes heart yin and
calms the spirit

Description: An Mien Pien is a mild
formula that possesses heart-nour-
ishing and heat-clearing properties.
In traditional Chinese medicine, the
heart is not only responsible for
blood circulation, it is also considered the "seat of the spirit." For this
reason, if the yin (nourishing
aspect) of the heart is depleted, the
person experiences anxiety, restlessness, and insomnia. This imbalance
in heart yin is treated with herbs
that are considered to "nourish the
heart and calm the spirit (shen)."
This category of herbs is repre-
sented in An Mien Pien by its two
chief ingredients: *Ziziphus* seed

(suan zao ren) and *Polygala* root
(yuan zhi). *Ziziphus* seeds have a
sedative, hypnotic, and analgesic
action and are indicated for insomnia, restlessness, and heart palpitations due to "deficiency of blood or
yin in the heart and liver."

Polygala root is another nourishing herb that calms the heart, making it useful for anxiety, restlessness,
insomnia, and disorientation.

Manufacturer: China National
Import and Export Corp.

Dosage: 4 tablets, three times a day

An Shen Bu Xin Wan

(ahn shen boo shin wahn);
"Peaceful Spirit Tonify
Heart Pill"

Indications: Insomnia, dizziness,
excessive dreaming, restlessness

Functions: Sedates the spirit, nourishes the heart and kidneys

Description: This formula is known

for its ability to calm anxiety, insomnia, excessive dreaming, and heart palpitations. Its chief ingredient is mother-of-pearl shell (zhen zhu mu), which is in the category of substances that "settle the heart and calm the spirit." Most of the members of this category are heavy sea shells and minerals, and they are meant to "anchor the spirit" in cases where the underlying deficiency of yin has allowed the yang (activity) to become relatively excessive. Typically, this yang excess produces more severe emotional imbalances than simple yin deficiency without extreme heat, and it requires a stronger tranquilizing effect than simple yin tonics that are mildly calming. Since the formula is composed of almost 50 percent mother-of-pearl shell, it can cause stomach irritation or indigestion in some individuals. In this event, it should be discontinued.

Manufacturer: Shanghai Native Medicine Works

Dosage: 15 pills, three times a day

Emperor's Tea, Tian Wang Bu Xin Dan (tyahn wahng boo shin dahn); "Emperor of Heaven's Pill to Tonify the Heart"

Indications: Insomnia, palpitations, anxiety, night sweats

Functions: Tonifies heart blood and yin, clears heat from deficiency

Description: This ancient formula in patent form is the classical remedy for the symptoms of "heart and kidney yin deficiency," an imbalance common in modern industrialized society. This type of depletion can occur from excessive mental work, improper diet, and "burning the candle at both ends." Symptoms include insomnia with restless sleep, disturbing dreams, anxiety, forgetfulness, mouth sores, inability to concentrate, and, possibly, night sweats. From a Western perspective, it can be used for mental or emotional disorders, insomnia, hypertension, menopause, or hyperthyroidism.

The chief herb is *Rehmannia glutinosa* (sheng di huang), chosen for its ability to replenish depleted reserves in the kidneys (yin essence). Substances that "nourish the heart and calm the spirit" are added, such as *Polygala tenuifolia* (yuan zhi), *Ziziphus spinosa* (suan zao ren), and *Biota orientalis* (bai zi ren). Another important ingredient is *Salvia miltiorrhiza* (dan shen), an important herb for treating palpitations, anxiety, and insomnia due to depletion of heart and kidney yin. Asparagus root (tian men dong) is added to increase the cooling, moistening actions of the formula. Finally, the formula contains *Schizandra* berries (wu wei zi). In addition to its ability to treat insomnia and palpitations due to depletion, *Schizandra* is considered an adaptogen similar to ginseng, meaning it may be capable of increasing the body's resistance to disease. It provides greater endurance and an improved capacity for dealing with stress. In the past, some versions of this patent were coated with a reddish powder called cinnabar. While this substance has strong sedative effects, it contains traces of mercury, a toxic heavy metal that is already too prevalent in modern industrialized countries. It is against the law to import cinnabar into the United States, so the mineral showed up only in patents that came through customs years before the ban. Telltale signs are a reddish color instead of the usual black pills, and the ingredient list includes cinnabar, known as zhu sha. It is worthwhile to be aware of the possibility, however remote, that patents with this coating may still be around. Therefore, check the color of the pills and the label on the bottle to be sure the patent you use is not coated with cinnabar.

Manufacturer: Lanzhou Foci

Dosage: 8 pills, three times a day. The formula should be taken for a few months to have a long-lasting effect.

Resources

National Organizations for Traditional Chinese Medicine

AMERICAN ASSOCIATION OF ORIENTAL MEDICINE
433 Front St.
Catasauqua, PA 18032
610–266–1433, fax: 610–264–2768
email: AAOM1@aol.com

NATIONAL ACUPUNCTURE AND ORIENTAL MEDICINE ALLIANCE
14637 Starr Rd. SE
Olalla, WA 98359
206–851–6896, fax: 206–851–6883
email: 76143.2061@compuserve.com

**NATIONAL CERTIFICATION COMMISSION
FOR ACUPUNCTURE AND ORIENTAL
MEDICINE (NCCA)**
P.O. Box 97075
Washington, DC 20090
202–232–1404, fax: 202–462–6157

Sources of Chinese Herb Seeds and Live Plants

ELIXIR BOTANICALS
General Delivery
Brixey, MO 65618
417–261–2393

HORIZON HERBS
P.O. Box 69
Williams, OR 97544
541–846–6704, fax: 541–846–6233

Chinese Healing Secrets

OREGON EXOTICS
1065 Messinger Rd.
Grants Pass, OR 97527
541–846–7578

RICHTERS
357 Highway 47
Goodwood, ON
Canada L0C 1A0
email: orderdesk@richters.com

Sources for Chinese Herbs and Extracts

EAST EARTH TRADE WINDS
P.O. Box 493151
Redding, CA 96049–3151
916–258–6878

MAYWAY CORPORATION
1338 Mandela Parkway
Oakland, CA 94607
510–208–3113, fax: 510–208–3069

MIN TONG HERBS / TASHI ENTERPRISES
322 7th St., #1
Oakland, CA 94607
800–538–1333, fax: 800–875–0798
Internet: www.tashi.com

Newsletter

HEALING FIELDS
P.O. Box 7256
Santa Cruz, CA 95061

Published quarterly, Healing Fields provides information about traditional Chinese medicine, research on herbs, therapeutic dietary recipes, and tips on strengthening the immune system and fighting disease. Cost: $25 per year.

Chinese Healing Secrets

Chinese Healing Secrets

INDEX